Easy Injections

Easy Injections

Lyn Weiss, MD, FAAPMR, FAANEM

Professor of Clinical Physical Medicine and Rehabilitation
SUNY-Stony Brook College of Medicine
Chairman and Program Director
Nassau University Medical Center, East Meadow, New York
Board Certified Physical Medicine and Rehabilitation
Board Certified Electrodiagnostic Medicine

Julie K. Silver, MD

Assistant Professor of Physical Medicine and Rehabilitation
Harvard Medical School, Boston, Massachusetts
Associate in Physiatry
Massachusetts General Hospital, Brigham and Women's Hospital, and Spaulding Rehabilitation Hospital, Boston, Massachusetts
Board Certified Physical Medicine and Rehabilitation

Ted A. Lennard, MD, FAAPMR

Clinical Assistant Professor, Department of Physical Medicine and Rehabilitation
University of Arkansas for Medical Sciences, Little Rock, Arkansas
Springfield Neurological and Spine Institute, Springfield, Missouri
Board Certified Physical Medicine and Rehabilitation

Jay M. Weiss, MD, FAAPMR, FAANEM

Assistant Professor of Clinical Physical Medicine and Rehabilitation
SUNY-Stony Brook College of Medicine
Board Certified Physical Medicine and Rehabilitation
Board Certified Electrodiagnostic Medicine
Board Certified Pain Medicine
NYS Certified Physician Acupuncturist

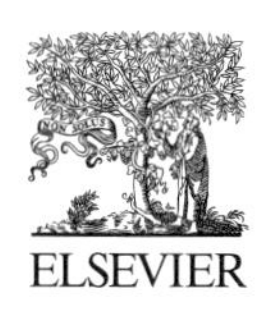

ELSEVIER

BUTTERWORTH
HEINEMANN
ELSEVIER

1600 John F. Kennedy Blvd.
Ste 1800
Philadelphia, PA 19103-2899

EASY INJECTIONS ISBN 978-0-7506-7527-7

Notice

Knowledge and best practice in this field are constantly changing. As new research and experience broaden our knowledge, changes in practice, treatment and drug therapy may become necessary or appropriate. Readers are advised to check the most current information provided (i) on procedures featured or (ii) by the manufacturer of each product to be administered, to verify the recommended dose or formula, the method and duration of administration, and contraindications. It is the responsibility of the practitioner, relying on their own experience and knowledge of the patient, to make diagnoses, to determine dosages and the best treatment for each individual patient, and to take all appropriate safety precautions. To the fullest extent of the law, neither the Publisher nor the Authors assume any liability for any injury and/or damage to persons or property arising out or related to any use of the material contained in this book.

The Publisher

Library of Congress Cataloging-in-Publication Data
Easy injections / Lyn Weiss ... [et al.]. – 1st ed.
p. ; cm.
Includes bibliographical references and index.
ISBN 978-0-7506-7527-7
1. Injections. 2. Musculoskeletal system–Diseases–Treatment. 3. Pain–Treatment.
I. Weiss, Lyn D. II. Title.
[DNLM: 1. Injections–methods. 2. Musculoskeletal Diseases–therapy. 3. Pain–therapy.
WB 354 E13 2007]
RM169.E47 2007
615′.6–dc22 2007023042

Acquisitions Editor: Susan F. Pioli
Developmental Editor: Joan Ryan
Senior Project Manager: David Saltzberg
Cover Designer: Steve Stave

Printed in the United States of America

Last digit is the print number: 9 8 7 6 5 4 3 2 1

Contents

	Dedication	ix
	Preface	xi
	Acknowledgments	xiii
1	Introduction to Injections	1
	Before You Get Started	*1*
	Postinjection Care	*4*
	Problems You May Encounter	*4*
2	Medications and Injection Supplies	8
	Introduction	*8*
	Medications	*8*
	Injection Supplies	*12*
	Conclusion	*13*
3	Joints	15
	Glenohumeral (Shoulder) Joint	*15*
	Acromioclavicular Joint	*19*
	Sternoclavicular Joint	*21*
	Elbow Joint	*23*
	Wrist Joint	*26*
	Intercarpal Joint	*29*
	First Carpometacarpal Joint	*31*
	Interphalangeal Joints	*34*
	Temporomandibular Joint	*36*
	Hip Joint	*39*
	Knee Joint	*43*
	Ankle Joint	*47*
	Subtalar Joint	*49*
	Intertarsal Joint	*53*
	Metatarsophalangeal Joint	*55*
4	Tendons	58
	Trigger Finger (Stenosing Flexor Tendosynovitis)	*58*
	De Quervain's (Tenosynovitis of the Wrist)	*61*
	Bicipital Tendinitis	*62*
	Lateral Epicondylitis	*66*

Medial Epicondylitis 69
Rotator Cuff Tendinitis 71
Plantar Fasciitis 74
Achilles Tendinitis 77
Iliotibial Band Tendinitis/Bursitis 79
Infrapatellar Tendinitis 82

5 Bursae 85
Subacromial Bursa (Subdeltoid Bursa) 85
Olecranon Bursa 87
Trochanteric Bursa 90
Ischial Bursa 92
Pes Anserine Bursa 95
Prepatellar Bursa 97
Achilles Bursa/Retrocalcaneal Bursa 100
Subcutaneous Achilles Bursa 102

6 Nerves 105
Suprascapular Nerve 105
Musculocutaneous Nerve 108
Greater and Lesser Occipital Nerve 110
Medial Antebrachial Cutaneous Nerve 113
Lateral Antebrachial Cutaneous Nerve 114
Radial Nerve Injection at the Elbow 118
Median Nerve Injection at the Wrist (Carpal Tunnel Injection) 121
Ulnar Nerve at Guyon's Canal 124
Iliohypogastric Nerve Block 127
Ilioinguinal Nerve Block 129
Lateral Femoral Cutaneous Nerve Injection (Meralgia Paresthetica Injection) 131
Obturator Nerve 134
Femoral Nerve 137
Saphenous Nerve Block 139
Tibial Nerve Injection (Tarsal Tunnel Injection) 142
Deep Peroneal Nerve Injection (Anterior Tarsal Tunnel) 145
Superficial Peroneal—Nerve Injection at the Ankle 148
Sural Nerve Block 150
Lower Extremity Digital Nerve Blocks 153

7 Trigger Point Injections 156
Mechanism of Action 156
Potential Risks 157

8 Botulinum Toxin 160
Mechanism of Action 160
Potential Risks 161
Botulinum Toxin Clinical Uses 162
Injection Procedure 162

9 Prolotherapy 166
Introduction *166*
History *166*
Mechanism of Action and Clinical Effectiveness *166*
Patient Selection *167*
Solutions Injected *167*
Injection Sites *168*
Injection Technique—Lumbar Spine Example *168*
Conclusion *170*

10 Acupuncture 172
Mechanism of Action *172*
Potential Risks *176*

11 Sympathetic Injections 178
Injection Anatomy of the Sympathetic System *178*
Complex Regional Pain Syndrome *179*
Patient Selection for Sympathetic Injections *180*
Cervical Stellate Ganglion Blocks CPT Code 64510 (Stellate Ganglion or Cervical Sympathetic) *180*
Lumbar Sympathetic Blocks CPT Code 64520 Lumbar or Thoracic (Paravertebral Sympathetics) *182*
Conclusions *183*

12 Spinal Injections 184
Patient Selection *184*
Who Is Qualified to Perform Spinal Injections? *185*
What Equipment Is Necessary? *185*
Potential Complications *185*
Spinal Injection Anatomy *187*
Loss of Resistance Technique *187*
Conclusion *200*

Index 201

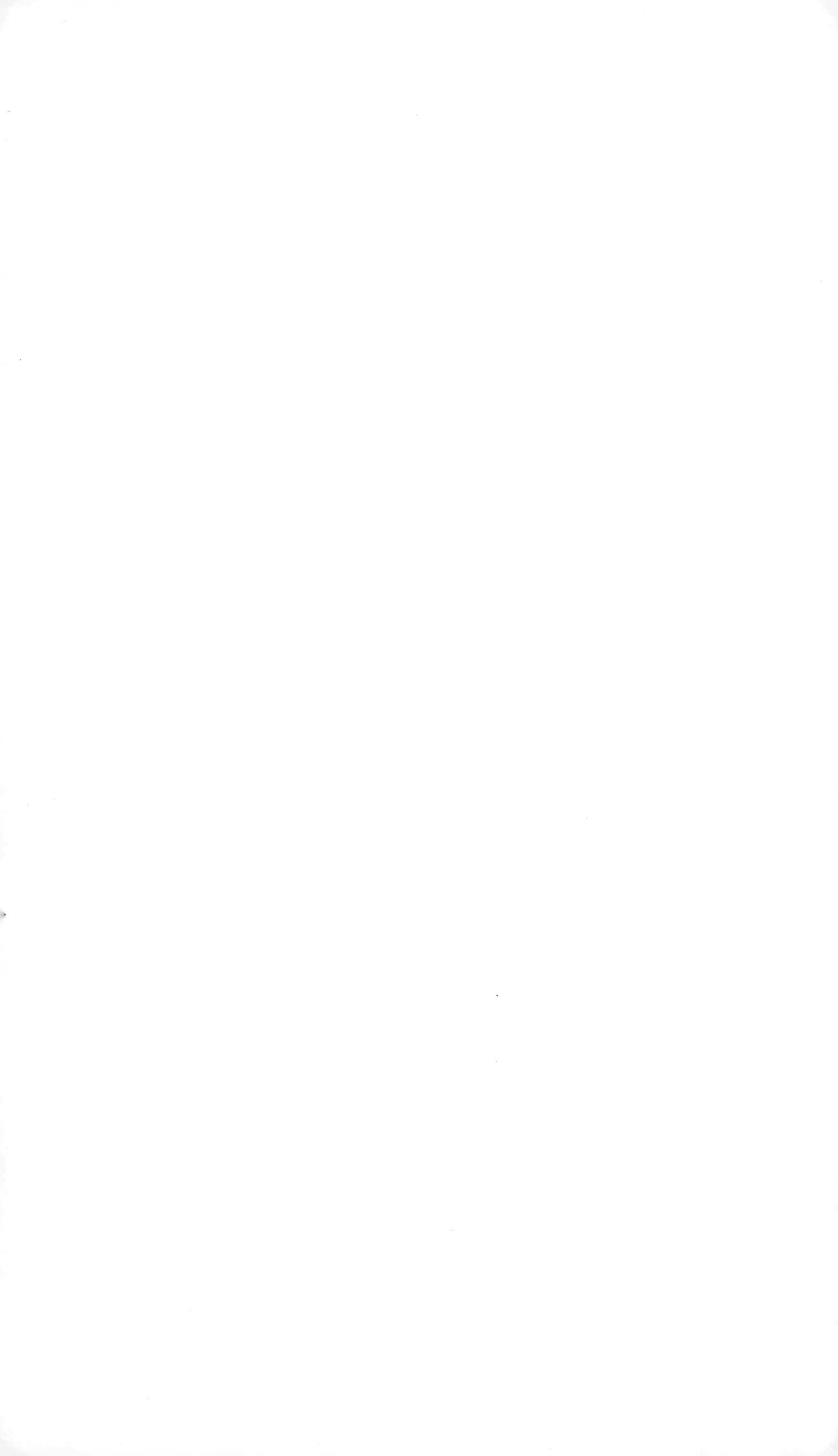

Dedication

This book is dedicated to our parents, our spouses, and our children (Ari, Helene, Stefan, Richie, Alex, Emily, Anna Rose, Suzanne, Selby, Claire, Julia, and Maura). It is also dedicated to our past, present, and future residents. We hope this book helps you become better physicians.

Preface

The injection procedures described here are based on a review of the various techniques described in the medical literature as well as the authors'experiences. The techniques chosen are thought to be the most appropriate in most cases. As clinical circumstances may differ, other approaches may be more appropriate for individual cases.

While this book describes technical procedures, it does not address the clinical decision making and the risk/benefit assessment that physicians must utilize in conjunction with these procedures. The reader is encouraged to familiarize him/herself with additional sources for additional approaches. In most cases, it will take preparation, practice, and mentoring before the physician can comfortably perform these procedures independently. As always, it is up to each physician to determine the most appropriate treatment for the patient. It is also up to that physician to assess his/her competence and ability to perform any procedure.

L. W.
J. K. S.
T. A. L.
J. M. W.

Acknowledgments

We would like to acknowledge the following people, who assisted in the preparation of this book:

Mary Alice Hanford
Dolores Meloni
Laura Anello
Sheila Slezak
Amanda Hellenthal
Susan Pioli
Joan Ryan
And special thanks to our models, Randi, Helene, and Stefan.

1

Introduction to Injections

Injections are procedures that cover many different therapeutic interventions. In this book, we are focusing on those injections that are used in treating painful musculoskeletal conditions. Injections are relatively straightforward to perform; however, they do take skill and practice. A healthcare practitioner who is an expert in performing pain injections follows these five basic rules:

1. Understand the anatomy where you are injecting.
2. Know the risks and benefits of the procedure.
3. Decide what medications, needles, and syringes you want to use.
4. Anticipate and be able to deal with adverse reactions.
5. Recommend appropriate postinjection care.

In this chapter, we will give you an overview of what you need to know to get started. Of course, this book does not take the place of mentoring from a skilled practitioner, but for the beginner, it provides a basis to understand how injections are done. Healthcare providers who are skilled at performing injections can use this book as an easy reference to quickly look up a wide variety of musculoskeletal procedures.

Before You Get Started

Know the Procedure You Want to Do

Before you inject a patient, you need to consider why you want to do an injection in the first place and how it may help (or potentially harm) the person. Basically, as with everything we do in medicine, you need to understand the benefit/risk profile. What are the benefits? What are the risks? The decision to do the injection, of course, is that the benefits greatly outweigh the risks. Injections performed by healthcare providers who are skilled have a very low rate of complications. Nevertheless, it is important to be very familiar with both the benefits and the risks involved.

Know Your Anatomy

This seems obvious, but it still is an important point to make. The more you know the anatomy around the area you plan to inject, the better you will be able to position your needle right where you want it to go (Table 1–1). We have provided pictures and diagrams in this book to help with this. A few important points must be remembered about anatomical placement. First, people are different, and they may not have the anatomy you are expecting. So, although it is important to know your anatomy, also consider common anatomical variations. In short, expect the unexpected. Second, patients will relax if you talk them through an injection, so think about how you want to position the patient for the

Table 1–1 How to Tell Where your Needle Is

Muscle: feels spongy and soft.
Tendon or ligament: feels fibrous and tough.
Capsule: often feels like pushing through a balloon where there is slight resistance and then you pop through to the other side.
Cartilage: feels sticky and tough.
Bone: is very hard and quite sensitive for the patient.

best access and then tell them why you are asking them to assume that position. This gives patients a sense that you know what you are doing, and this, in turn, will help them relax. Third, no matter how confident you are that your needle is in the right place, it is important to *aspirate* (Table 1–2). None of the injections described in this book should be done into a blood vessel. So be sure and draw the needle back a bit before you inject.

Decide on the Equipment You Will Need

The equipment you choose is very important. A needle with a too-large diameter will cause unnecessary pain. On the other hand, a needle with a too-small diameter will not allow the injected materials to pass through. In the next chapter, we describe the various types of medications, needles, and syringes. It is also essential that you incorporate aseptic techniques into your procedures (Table 1–3). Infection is a real risk to the patient (although the incidence for all these injections when done properly is very low), and it is important to minimize this as much as possible.

Table 1–2 Aspirates

1. Frank blood: Usually there is a history of recent trauma and joint swelling. Aspirating the blood provides significant pain relief, allows the joint to be more mobile, and removes an irritant that causes synovitis. Because of the history of trauma, it is essential to be sure to get an x-ray and rule out a concomitant fracture. It is also a good idea to keep in mind that if there is a hemarthrosis in the knee, 40% of the time there is an associated anterior cruciate ligament (ACL) rupture.[1]
2. Serous fluid: This colorless or pale yellow fluid signals a noninflammatory process. It is fine to inject a joint with serous fluid aspirate; however, if you have any doubts, send the aspirate to the laboratory before you inject any drugs into the joint. It is not uncommon to have this streaked with blood, and this is usually related to the trauma of the procedure itself.
3. Xanthochromic fluid: This orange-colored fluid is due to old blood that has broken down. The presence of this fluid implies a history of trauma.
4. Turbid fluid: This fluid appears darker and more turbid than normal fluid (because of an increase in cells and debris) and signals infection, although it is not always easy to identify. Any time you suspect infection, send the aspirate for microscopic and culture examination in the laboratory. If you suspect gout or pseudogout, send the aspirate for crystal analysis.
5. Frank pus: This is rare in an outpatient setting. A patient with an aspirate that demonstrates frank pus (which often has a foul smell) is likely to be extremely ill and requires hospitalization.
[1]Saunders, Stephanie. Injection Techniques in Orthopaedic Practice. Second edition. W.B. Saunders, London, 2002, page 17.

Table 1–3 Aseptic Technique

1. Use prepackaged sterile disposable needles and syringes.
2. Use only single-dose medication vials when possible.
3. Change needles after drawing up the solution into the syringe (i.e., do not use the same needle to inject the patient as the one you used to draw up the drugs).
4. Wear gloves. It is best if you can wear sterile, nonlatex type.
5. Clean the skin with alcohol, povidone iodine (Betadine), or other sterilizing preparations.
6. Do not touch the site after you clean it (this includes touching the site with your finger to guide the needle).
7. Always aspirate, but, particularly for joints, be sure that the aspirate does not appear infected.

It is important to stock not only the equipment you need for the procedure but also any equipment you may need in an emergency situation. This equipment may include:

Emergency Basics

- Disposable plastic airways
- Ambu bag/mask
- Epi-Pen or adrenaline 1:1000 strength

Protect Yourself and the Patient

It is advisable for anyone performing injections to be vaccinated for Hepatitis B. Other precautions include always wearing gloves and sometimes a gown and/or mask.

Performing an Injection

To perform an injection well, you do need to practice. Watching someone else do it is important for beginners. When you are ready to perform the procedure yourself, follow these simple guidelines:

- Prepare the patient by explaining the procedure in detail, including the risks and benefits, and obtain written informed consent. Be sure to document the risks on the consent form.
- Place the patient in the optimal position.
- Organize your medications and equipment.
- Mark your site with an object that will not pierce the skin (e.g., clean finger nail, needle guard).
- Clean the skin and allow it to dry.
- Don your gloves and draw up your medications.
- Use a fresh needle to inject.
- Pierce the skin and direct the needle to your target.
- Aspirate.
- Inject (be sure there is no evidence of infection).

One tip for aspirating: when you are finished aspirating, unscrew the syringe with the needle still in place (making sure not to touch the back end of the needle hub to maintain aseptic technique) and then screw on a new syringe filled with the medications you plan to inject. This allows you to do two procedures, aspiration and injection, with one needle stick.

Postinjection Care

Postinjection care is very important but will vary depending on the type of injection performed. After the injection, some type of sterile adhesive dressing (a simple band-aid is often fine) should be applied. In general, it is advisable to have patients stay in the office for at least 20–30 minutes after the injection to be sure no immediate complications, such as allergic reactions or bleeding, develop. Some practitioners will opt to place an ice pack on the injected site for a portion of this time (do not ice an area for more than 15–20 minutes). The patient can be advised to ice at home for 15–20 minutes, with several hours between each ice pack treatment. For more details on postinjection care, refer to the specific injections in this book.

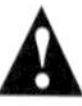

Problems You May Encounter

Injection issues usually fall into one of the following categories:

- Problems with the medication selection or dose.
- Problems with the needle size.
- Injecting into the wrong area.
- Poor injection technique.
- Adverse patient reactions to the medication or the procedure itself.
- Lack of proper postinjection care and rehabilitation.

Problems with the Medication Selection or Dose

Problems with the medication selection or dose are easy to understand but are not always so easy to avoid. As is explained in the next chapter, no rigid standards exist for choosing injectable drugs. We provide some guidelines and tips in this text, but a few hard and fast rules should be followed. Carefully read each section before performing that type of injection for more information on drugs and dosing. When corticosteroids are being used, it is helpful to recognize that although the injections may be repeated (a general guideline is that they may be repeated up to three times in 1 year with at least 4–6 weeks in between injections), if the patient does not respond at all to the first injection, it is far less likely that he/she will respond to subsequent injections (unless the first injection failed because the medication did not reach its target). Usually, repeat injections are done for those who respond initially but continue to have symptoms or their symptoms recur. Another important point to consider is that the International Olympic Committee Medical Commission does list local anesthetics and corticosteroids as Class III drugs, which are subject to certain restrictions. If you are not the team doctor but are considering an injection in an athlete, it is best to discuss this with the team physician and follow the proper procedures for getting clearance.

Problems with the Needle Size

As mentioned earlier, the diameter of the needle is important. You want to choose the smallest diameter in which the drug (or aspirate) will easily flow. The length of the needle is also important. Too short a needle may prohibit you from being able to get the tip of the needle where you want it. With too long a needle, you may not have ideal control.

Long needles make it easier to inject tissues that you would not ordinarily reach (e.g., a too long needle in a trigger point injection in the upper back may cause a pneumothorax if it punctures the lung). Also, there have been instances of needles breaking off during injections, so you want to have the best control possible and definitely not place excessive stress on the needle.

Injecting into the Wrong Area

Most of the time when you inject into the wrong area, you do not harm the patient, but the injection will not work. However, it is certainly possible to inject the wrong area and cause harm as was mentioned in the previous example with the pneumothorax.

Poor Injection Technique

Sometimes the only result of poor injection technique is that the patient experiences more pain than he/she would if a more skilled practitioner had performed the procedure. Keeping in mind that all of these procedures are done to alleviate pain, it stands to reason that it is absolutely essential to inflict as little pain as possible on the patient during an injection. Poor technique can also result in other problems, such injecting the wrong target, unnecessary spread of medication to adjacent tissues, and too many or too few injections. Good technique comes with skill and practice; however, if you choose the right size needle, you know your anatomy, and you place the patient in the proper position, you will have done a lot to ensure proper technique before you even pierce the skin.

Adverse Patient Reactions to the Medication or the Procedure Itself

There are two main types of adverse reactions that may occur within seconds or minutes of injecting someone. These are listed as follows:

1. Syncopal or near syncopal events: This reaction usually occurs when people are anxious or fearful; however, it may occur without warning in a patient who seems perfectly calm. Feeling light-headed or fainting is not a result of the medication but rather of having the procedure itself. Patients will often tell you that they do not feel well and may offer specific symptoms such as feeling sweaty, nauseous, light-headed, or ringing in the ears. This is a sympathetic nervous system reaction, so the patient may appear pale and have bradycardia and hypotension. If you suspect someone may react this way during an injection (because of either a history of syncopal episodes or because of current anxiety), take extra time to be reassuring and place him/her in a position where he/she is lying down if possible. If this reaction happens during the injection, abort the procedure and have the patient lie down. Talk to the patient and be very reassuring. Patients who faint will usually recover within a minute or so, and they rarely have incontinence (compared with patients who have seizures that generally last longer and are often associated with incontinence); 35% oxygen may be given to a patient who has fainted.
2. Anaphylaxis: This is the most dreaded complication of an injection and fortunately is very rare. Anaphylaxis occurs when someone is highly allergic to a given medication and usually occurs within a few minutes of receiving the drug. No history of an allergy may be present. Symptoms may include flushing, itchy skin or rash, nausea/vomiting, abdominal pain, feeling drunk or confused, tachycardia, convulsions, facial or angioedema, breathing difficulties, or respiratory depression. Circulatory collapse, cardiac arrest, and death may follow. Immediate action can be lifesaving and includes using an Epi-Pen or some other form of adrenaline

Table 1–4 Contraindications to Injections

1. Infection near the site or sepsis is an absolute contraindication.
2. Known hypersensitivity or allergic reaction to a medication is an absolute contraindication.
3. Acute fracture is an absolute contraindication.
4. Children: Injections are very rare in children younger than 18 and should only be pursued with good reason after other treatments have failed.
5. Recent trauma: Unless you are aspirating blood from a joint, usually injections are not done immediately after trauma because this may cause more damage.
6. Prosthetic joint: Injections are usually not recommended around prosthetic joints.
7. Diabetic patients: May have a higher incidence of infection, and corticosteroids may temporarily elevate blood sugar levels.
8. Anticoagulation: People taking anticoagulants should be injected with caution. A skilled practitioner who avoids excessive trauma with the needle and applies additional pressure after the injection can usually do this safely. However, if the international normalized ratio (INR) is elevated, it is wise to avoid injecting someone who is anticoagulated until the INR is in the proper range.
9. Immunocompromised: Care should be taken when considering injecting anyone who is immunocompromised because of the increased risk of infection.
10. Anxiety: People who are anxious or fearful of injections should not have them unless there is a very good reason to proceed.

(1 mL of subcutaneous or intramuscular adrenaline 1:1000 may be given). It is crucial to maintain the airway, give cardiopulmonary resuscitation, if necessary, and summon help.

Other reactions that may also occur within hours, days, or even weeks of having had an injection (Table 1–4) are listed as follows:

1. Postinjection pain flare: This occurs in the range of 2–10% of the time and is most commonly seen with soft tissue injections.[2] This is a wheal-and-flare reaction, and usually no treatment is required, except perhaps a cold pack for 10–20 minutes. If the patient is uncomfortable, topical over-the-counter creams or lotions may help. If symptoms persist, occasionally an oral antihistamine is warranted.
2. Subcutaneous atrophy or skin depigmentation: Depigmentation occurs with corticosteroids and is more common when the injection is superficial and the patient has dark skin. Repeat injections may also make this more likely to occur. Atrophy of subcutaneous tissue or, for example, the fat pad in the heel with a plantar fasciitis injection may pose considerable long-term problems for the patient.
3. Bleeding or bruising may occur at or near the injection site.
4. Nerve damage may occur if the needle hits a nerve (shocklike pain is characteristic).

[2]Saunders, Stephanie. Injection Techniques in Orthopaedic Practice. Second edition. W. B. Saunders, London, 2002, page 6.

5. Steroid "chalk" may be found at previously injected sites, including around tendons or in the carpal tunnel. It is not known whether there is any clinical significance to these deposits.
6. Corticosteroids may be chondrotoxic (toxic to cartilage) and, therefore, should be undertaken with caution in joints. These drugs may also cause the weakening of tendons, although this is somewhat controversial. For this reason, it is usually not advisable to inject in or around the Achilles tendon (this weight-bearing tendon may be particularly susceptible to rupture, and it is generally accepted to avoid injections in this region).
7. Infection or sepsis is very rare but may occur. A red area around the injected area may be mistaken for infection when, in fact, it is a postinjection flare. If an infection is suspected, look for other evidence such as fever, elevated leukocyte count, or positive aspirate tissue culture.

After reading this chapter, you now know the basic principles that may be applied to all injections. In the next chapter, we will discuss how to choose the right medications, needles, and syringes. Then, we will go directly to specific injection types that make up the remainder of this text.

2

Medications and Injection Supplies

Introduction

This chapter will review common medications injected into the spine, joints, soft tissue, and tendon sheaths. These medications include corticosteroids and anesthetics and are commonly used by most physicians who treat any type of painful disorders associated with the musculoskeletal system. A brief discussion about vasoconstrictor agents and hyaluronic acid is also contained in this chapter. In addition to medications, this chapter will briefly discuss injection supplies required for most office-based or spinal injections.

Medications

Most injections used to treat painful conditions consist of a mixture of corticosteroids and anesthetics. This combination allows the patient to experience immediate anesthesia within the area injected while receiving the corticosteroid's anti-inflammatory effect on injured tissue over the next few days to weeks. A physician's preference of which specific anesthetic and corticosteroid to inject, in part, depends on the specific needs of the patient and whether or not a clear diagnosis has been established. For example, a single combined corticosteroid and anesthetic first dorsal compartment injection may be indicated for the patient with a clear diagnosis of de Quervain's tenosynovitis with a short-acting corticosteroid (e.g., triamcinolone) and a short-acting anesthetic (e.g., 1% lidocaine). If the patient does not respond to this injection, one may consider an anesthetic-only superficial radial sensory block with 2% lidocaine. The purpose of this injection would be to monitor the response to identify the possible pain generators within the thumb and radial side of the distal forearm. Other injectables such as normal saline or sterile water can be used when one needs to expand the volume injected without risking possible side effects such as anesthetic toxicity. This is more commonly performed when caudal epidural injections are given and large volumes of injectate are required.

Glucocorticosteroids

Glucocorticosteroids are often referred to as corticosteroids, "steroids," or "cortisone" by both the medical community and lay persons. They are frequently misunderstood by the public, who view these medications as both harmful and to be feared. These feelings are fueled, in part, by their confusion of the side effects known to exist with illegal androgenic steroids. These side effects are well publicized in the media and, most notably, include muscle hypertrophy, hair growth, and aggressive behaviors. Glucocorticosteroids can be differentiated from these androgenic steroids on the basis of their primary mode of action—the anti-inflammatory effect.

In general, corticosteroids produced by the adrenal cortex can be classified as androgenic or estrogenic, salt retaining (mineralocorticoids), and anti-inflammatory (glucocorticoids). The glucocorticoid class is commonly used in injections for the treatment of painful inflammatory disorders. The primary glucocorticoid produced in humans is cortisol (hydrocortisone). Cortisol and other synthetic glucocorticoids possess varying degrees of anti-inflammatory and salt-retaining properties. These are the properties that dictate which glucocorticoid should be injected (Table 2–1).

Side Effects

Side effects of glucocorticoids depend on the dosage and duration of treatment. Short-term use is commonly associated with reversible side effects and can be divided into two general categories—local and systemic. Common local side effects include skin and subcutaneous atrophy, periarticular atrophy, hair loss at the injection site, and alterations in skin pigmentation. These findings can be dramatic, especially in dark-skinned individuals. One need only to observe this side effect in patients to realize the alarming cosmetic changes possible from a single injection. To reduce these risks, the practitioner should be conscious of the potency and dosage of the glucocorticoid used and the depth at which the medication is injected. This cosmetic risk can also be reduced by flushing a needle with anesthetic or sterile water before removing it from the injection site to prevent a "steroid trail." Other local reactions that can be found in the literature include cartilage and tendon attrition, crystal-induced arthritis, and pericapsular calcification. Animal studies have demonstrated the adverse affects of intratendinous (i.e., injecting directly into a tendon) corticosteroid on the biomechanical properties of tendons (Kapetanos, 1982; Ketchum, 1971). Corticosteroids may alter or inhibit the formation of granulation, adhesions, or connective tissue; reduce tendon size; and reduce the biomechanical load that can be sustained before tendon failure. The effects of peritendinous (i.e., injecting into the region surrounding a tendon) corticosteroid injections in humans are not well established; however, a review of the literature reveals that numerous case reports of tendon rupture exist (Gottlieb and Riskin, 1980; Nichols, 2005; Unverfirth and Olix, 1973).

Systemic complications of corticosteroids can occur in most organ systems. Common reversible reactions include facial flushing, mood swings, tachycardia, hypertension, anxiety, hyperglycemia, gastrointestinal bleed, congestive heart failure, glaucoma,

Table 2–1 Glucocorticoid Anti-inflammatory Potency* (Lennard, 1995)

Hydrocortisone (cortisol)	1
Cortisone	0.8
Prednisone	4–5
Prednisolone	4–5
Methylprednisolone (Medrol, Depo-Medrol)	5
Triamcinolone (Aristocort, Kenalog)	5
Betamethasone	25–30
Dexamethasone (Decadron)	25–30

*Relative to hydrocortisone.

pancreatitis, myopathies, and increased appetite. Long-term affects from chronic treatment may include cataracts, aseptic necrosis of bone, amenorrhea, hyperlipidemia, muscle weakness, cushingoid appearance, osteoporosis, and suppression of the hypothalamic pituitary adrenal axis.

Anesthetics

Most physicians are familiar with common anesthetics, particularly those in the "caine" family, such as lidocaine or Marcaine. These drugs allow for the reduction or elimination of sensation from a joint, tendon, or nerve and provide temporary anesthesia. This change in their condition assists the physician in determining the tissue pain generator, thus helping with a diagnosis. More commonly, these drugs are used before surgical procedures.

There are two common classes of anesthetics: esters and amides (Table 2–2). These two general classes can be differentiated on the basis of their different bonding or linkage characteristics between the hydrophilic and lipophilic rings of the anesthetic molecule. This bonding defines the chemical properties observed with each of these classes of anesthetics.

Ester Anesthetics

Ester anesthetics have an ester linkage between these two rings that is hydrolyzed rapidly by the plasma enzyme cholinesterase. This results in short half-lives of these anesthetics. Their metabolites, which include paraaminobenzoic acid (PABA), are eliminated largely unchanged in the urine. Ester anesthetics possess a small, but possible, allergic reaction potential.

Amide Anesthetics

Amide anesthetics have an amide linkage between the lipophilic and hydrophilic portion of the anesthetic molecule. These drugs are hydrolyzed by liver enzymes to inactive metabolites and excreted in the urine. Approximately one third of these drugs can be excreted unchanged in the urine. Patients with abnormal hepatic blood flow, such as those with congestive heart failure or hepatic enzyme disorders, are at higher risk of toxicity. In general, amide anesthetics have a very low incidence of allergic reactions and are thought to be safer than ester anesthetics.

Side Effects

Anesthetic side effects are dose related. They frequently result from rapid absorption from the injection site or from a direct vascular injection. Many believe their risk of toxicity is better correlated with concentrations within the regional venous drainage systems

Table 2–2 Common Anesthetics

Esters
Procaine (Novocain)
Tetracaine
Chloroprocaine
Amides
Lidocaine
Bupivicaine
Mepivacaine
Etidocaine

(Mather *et al.*, 2005); sudden abnormal increases in their plasma levels result in toxicity. Table 2–3 lists the maximum doses of commonly used amide anesthetics. These maximum doses vary, depending on comorbid medical conditions and the route and speed of administration. These dose ranges serve only as guidelines, and each physician should establish proper doses for individual patients.

Toxicity manifests itself most commonly systemically and usually involves two organ systems, cardiovascular and neurological. One should be cautious in dosing anesthetics in patients with renal, hepatic, and cardiac diseases because dosage should be reduced. The magnitude of the reduction should be related to the expected influence of the pharmacodynamic change (Rosenberg *et al.*, 2004).

Anesthetic complications are dose related and involve the cardiovascular and neurological systems

Cardiovascular Complications

Anesthetics interfere with the electrical and mechanical activity of the myocardium and can be considered direct myocardial depressants. This can occur with abnormal plasma levels that may prolong both the QRS and PR intervals and cause significant hypotension. Furthermore, bradycardia, arrhythmias, angina, and cardiac arrest can occur. Bupivacaine, especially, requires caution in use during pregnancy or in cases of hypoxemia because it slowly disassociates from myocardium, causing prolonged myocardial depression.

Central Nervous System Complications

Central nervous system manifestations of toxicity are directly related to the degree of plasma elevation of the specific anesthetic. At lower plasma levels (3–5 μg/mL), one may experience anxiety, dizziness, light-headedness, metallic taste in the mouth, circumoral or tongue numbness, and tinnitus. In moderate plasma levels (8 μg/mL), muscular twitching or tremors, visual and auditory disturbances, nausea, and slurred speech may occur. In levels ≥10–12 μg/mL, drowsiness, hallucinations, seizures, and coma are seen.

Vasoconstrictor Agents

Vasoconstrictor agents can be used to reduce local tissue bleeding. The vascular constriction provided by these agents also reduces absorption of the anesthetic and prolongs anesthesia.

Table 2–3 Comparison of Common Amide Anesthetics

	Onset	Duration* (min)	Equal (min)	Toxicity**	Max† dose mg/kg
Lidocaine	0.5–1	100	1	5	4.5–5.0
Bupivacaine	5	120–240	0.25	2	2.0‡
Mepivacaine	3–5	100	1	4	7.0§
Etidocaine	5	120–240	0.25	3	4.0–6.0

*Varies with method of administration.

**Toxicity comparison (1, most toxic, 7, least toxic).

†Dose listed is without epinephrine.

‡Maximum dose is 120–170 mg.

§Maximum dose is 400 mg.

This allows for the use of lower concentrations of anesthetics and, therefore, reduces the risk of toxicity. The most commonly used vasoconstrictor is epinephrine in concentrations of 1:100,000–1:200,000. The use of vasoconstrictors may cause increased injection pain, increased wound infection, and increases in the risk of tissue necrosis in the digits, ears, nose, and penis. Systemic symptoms such as tachycardia, angina, anxiety, tremors, dizziness, headaches, hypertension, palpitations, and arrhythmias are also possible.

Hyaluronic Acid

Hyaluronic acid is an elastoviscous fluid containing hylan polymers that are derivatives of hyaluronan, a naturally occurring complex sugar. Cells in the cartilage of joints secrete this naturally occurring substance. Hyaluronan is one of the major molecular components of synovial fluid and gives this fluid its viscous, slippery quality. The high viscosity of synovial fluid provides for a smooth gliding surface for joints to articulate. Hyaluronic acid has been approved for the treatment of osteoarthritis of the knee joint for viscosupplementation in patients who have failed to respond adequately to conservative therapy. This substance is given in the form of weekly injections into the knee joint over a 15-day period for a total of three injections.

Various drugs now exist to promote viscosupplementation and include Synvisc (hylan), Hyalgan (sodium hyaluronate), Orthovisc (high molecular weight hyaluronan), Artz (sodium hyaluronate), and Euflexxa (1% sodium hyaluronate). Few contraindications have been reported as a result of the medication other than hypersensitivity to hyaluronan products, allergies to avian proteins, lactating females, children, and pregnancy.

Injection Supplies

The supplies necessary for most injections are usually present in most physician offices.

For spinal procedures, additional needles and equipment would be required. Following is a list of commonly used supplies.

Common Injection Supplies

Needles

Medication Aspiration

18-gauge, 1¼ inch
20-gauge, 1¼ inch

Skin Anesthesia

27-gauge 1¼ inch
30-gauge 1¼ inch

Soft Tissue or Joint Injections

22-gauge 1¼ or 3½ inch
25-gauge 1¼ or 3½ inch

Spinal Injections

22-gauge 3½-inch spinal needle
25-gauge 3½-inch spinal needle

18-gauge 3½-inch Tuohy needle
20-gauge 3½-inch Tuohy needle

Syringes

6-cc plastic syringe, Luer lock
12-cc plastic syringe, Luer lock
2- or 5-cc glass syringes for epidurals with loss of resistance technique

Skin Antiseptics

Alcohol pads
Betadine
Hibiclens

Miscellaneous

Band-Aids
Gloves—sterile and nonsterile
Skin markers
Sterile and nonsterile 2 × 2 or 4 × 4 sponges
Sterile drapes
Tubing

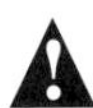

Conclusion

The proper selection of medications and the knowledge of anesthetic or corticosteroid dosing are, in part, responsible for the success or failure of an injection. Corticosteroids must be used judiciously, and the practitioner should be aware of the potential problems these medications possess. The practitioner must also be keenly aware of dose-related complications from anesthetics and be able to manage these problems when they occur. These complications most often affect the cardiovascular and neurological systems. Along with medications, an overview of injection supplies, which are typically found in most physician offices, has been given.

REFERENCES

Gottlieb, N. L., and Riskin, W. G. (1980). Complications of local corticosteroid injections. *JAMA* **240,** 1547–1548.

Kapetanos, G. (1982). The effect of the local corticosteroids on the healing and biomechanical properties of the partially injured tendon. *Clin. Orthop.* **163,** 170–179.

Ketchum, L. D. (1971). Effects of triamcinolone on tendon healing and function. *Plast. Reconstr. Surg.* **47,** 471.

Lennard, T. A. (1995). Fundamentals of procedural care. *In* "Physiatric Procedures in Clinical Practice." (T. A. Lennard, Ed.), Philadelphia, Hanley & Belfus.

Mather, L. E., Compeland, S. E., and Ladd, L. A. (2005). Acute toxicity of local anesthetics: Underlying pharmacokinetic and pharmacodynamic concepts. *Reg. Anesth. Pain Med* **30(6),** 553–566.

Nichols, A.W. (2005). Complications associated with the use of corticosteroids in the treatment of athletic injuries. *Clin. J. Sport. Med.* **15(5),** E370.

Rosenberg, P. H., Veering, B. T., and Urmey, W. F. (2004). Maximum recommended doses of local anesthetics: A multifactorial concept. *Reg. Anesth. Pain Med.* **29(6),** 524–575.

Unverfirth, L. J., and Olix, M. L. (1973). The effect of local steroid injections on tendon. *J. Bone Joint Surg. (Am)* **55,** 1315.

3

Joints

The injection procedures here are based on a review of the various techniques described in the medical literature as well as the authors' experiences. The techniques chosen are felt to be the most appropriate in most cases. As clinical circumstances may differ, other approaches may be more appropriate for individual cases. The reader is encouraged to familiarize himself/herself with the additional sources in the bibliography at the end of this chapter for additional approaches.

All procedures should be performed using appropriate preparation and aseptic technique. Local anesthesia (either injected or vapo-coolant spray) may be helpful in most procedures. As always, the clinician should weigh the risks and benefits of any interventional procedure.

Glenohumeral (Shoulder) Joint

Name of Procedure

Intraarticular injection of the glenohumeral joint is the name of this procedure.

CPT

The Current Procedural Terminology code is 20610 (injection of major joint).

Indications

Intraarticular injections of the glenohumeral joint are usually performed for pain caused by arthritis (most commonly osteoarthritis secondary to trauma) or adhesive capsulitis (also known as "frozen shoulder"). Injection is usually offered after a patient has had a course of NSAIDs and/or physical therapy (including weighted pendulum stretching and isometric strengthening of the external rotator and muscles of abduction) fail and before surgery (debridement of the glenohumeral joint or joint replacement) is considered. The injection can be diagnostic (to help differentiate shoulder pain caused by joint disease versus rotator cuff diseases). Intraarticular injection may be combined with capsular dilation (which involves injecting saline to help create more space in the joint and break up adhesions) for adhesive capsulitis.

Symptoms

- Pain and stiffness localized to the shoulder. Pain may be felt in the forearm or deltoid region.
- Pain worse with activity and all shoulder movements.
- Decreased functional status secondary to pain and decreased range of motion.

Physical Examination Findings

- Decreased active and passive range of motion of the shoulder, especially external rotation and abduction (in contrast, with rotator cuff pathology, including tears, only active motion is usually affected).
- Crepitus may be noted on range of motion.
- Tenderness may be noted over the anterior rotator cuff and the posterior joint line.
- May see wasting of surrounding shoulder muscles caused by disuse.

Medications to Inject

Corticosteroid and local anesthetic mixture is used for injection. Some physicians prefer injecting hyaluronic acid.

Amount to Inject

The amount for injection is 3–4 mL (more for hydraulic distention with normal saline for adhesive capsulitis).

Size and Gauge of Needle

A 1½-inch 22-gauge needle is used. The length of the needle will depend on how much subcutaneous tissue is in the affected area.

Local Anatomy

The glenohumeral joint lies between the articular cartilage of the glenoid labrum and the humeral head. For the anterior approach, the coracoid process and the medial humeral head should be located and marked. For the posterior approach, the lateral and posterior acromion should be located and marked. The posterolateral point of the acromion should be identified.

Patient Position

The patient is seated with the arm in the lap with the shoulder slightly internally rotated.

How and Where to Inject

An anterior or posterior approach may be used (Figures 3–1 to 3–4).

Anterior Approach

For the anterior approach (see Figures 3–1 and 3–2), insert the needle ½ inch below the coracoid process and medial to the head of the humerus. Direct the needle outward and

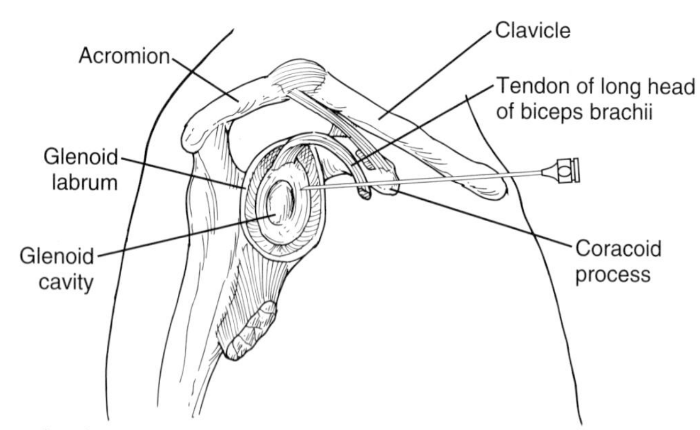

Fig 3–1 Glenohumeral joint injection—anterior approach.

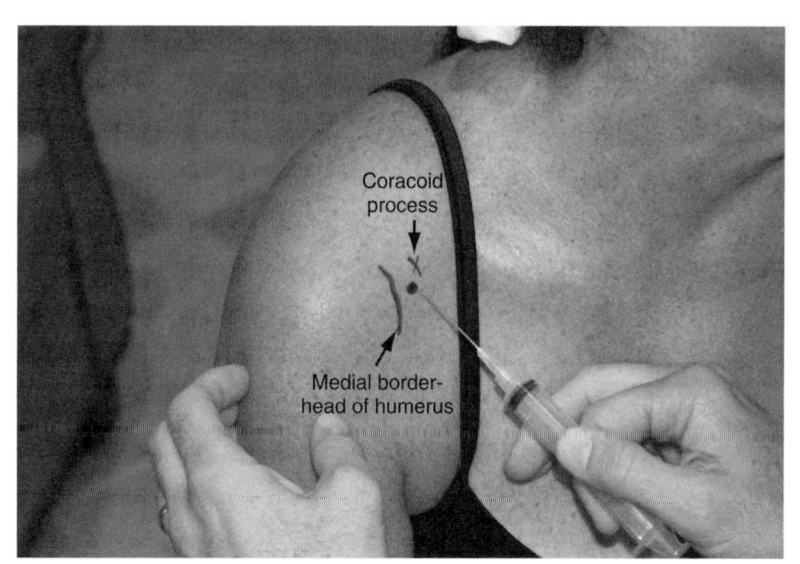

Fig 3–2 Glenohumeral joint injection—anterior approach.

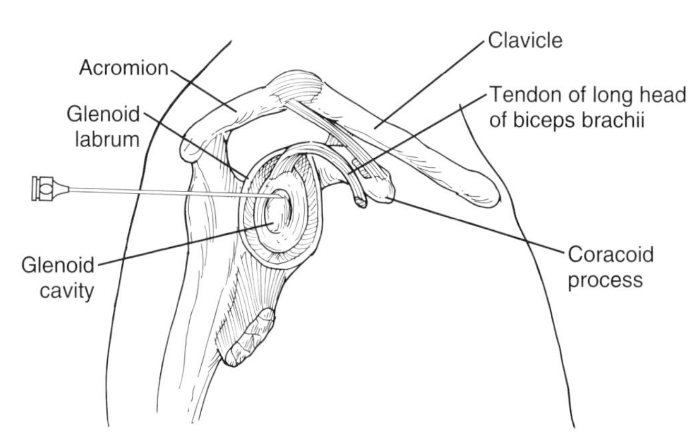

Fig 3–3 Glenohumeral joint injection—posterior approach

upward toward the medial portion of the humeral head. When the needle hits the bone (humeral head), the needle is withdrawn slightly into the joint space. There should be little resistance to injection if the needle is in the joint. If there is resistance, the needle may be in a ligament or tendon, and the position should be changed. Aspirate the joint before injecting to avoid intravascular injection and to ensure that gross signs of infection are not present.

Posterior Approach

In the posterior approach (see Figures 3–3 and 3–4), the needle is inserted approximately 1 cm under the posterolateral angle of the acromion (see Figure 3–2). The needle is directed anteriorly and medially toward the coracoid process. The needle should be horizontal because if it is directed upward, it may enter the subacromial space instead of the joint space. When the needle hits the bone, the needle is withdrawn slightly into the joint space. There should be little resistance to injection if the needle is in the joint. If there is resistance, the needle may be in a

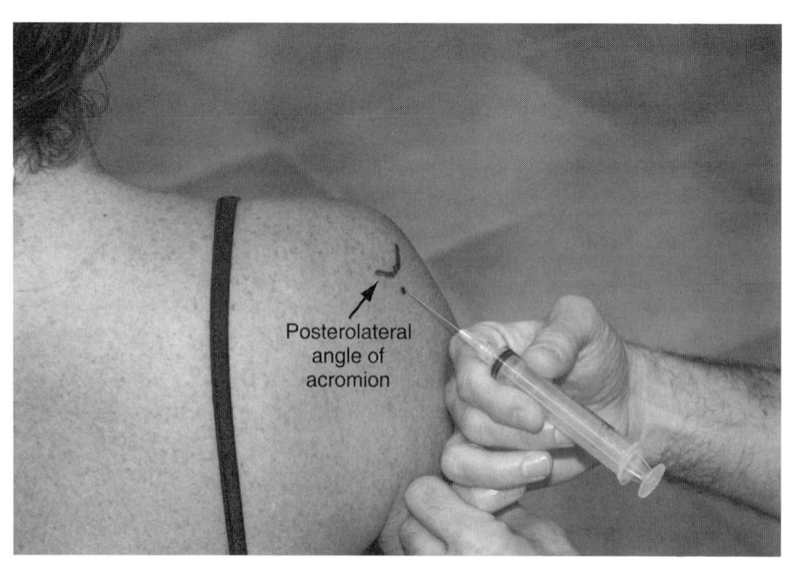

Fig 3–4 Glenohumeral joint injection—posterior approach.

ligament or tendon, and the position should be changed. Aspirate the joint before injecting to avoid intravascular injection and to ensure that gross signs of infection are not present.

Pitfalls/Complications

X-rays should be taken of the joint before injection. Do not inject the joint if acute infection is suspected. It is anticipated that the patient may have an increase in pain for a few days caused by the use of corticosteroids. Informing patients of this helps to alleviate their postinjection pain concerns. If there is no relief from the injection, consider other sources of pain (rotator cuff tear, fractures, bursitis, tendinitis, pseudogout, neoplasm, avascular necrosis, rheumatoid arthritis, infection). Many of these diagnoses can be ruled out by a standard set of x-rays. Further imaging such as MRI or CT scans may be warranted if the x-rays are unrevealing and the patient does not respond to an injection or a series of injections. The risk of infection can be minimized with sterile preparation of the area and aseptic technique. Bursitis and/or tendinitis may coexist and may require additional treatment.

Postinjection Care

Apply a sterile dressing and pressure over the injection site. Have the patient ice the affected area for 20 minutes two to three times daily for the first 24–48 hours. Then begin local heat and gentle stretching exercises several days after the injection. Avoid vigorous exercise or overhead activities for several days.

When to Perform Follow-Up Injections

Although there are no strict guidelines, a reasonable approach is to reinject in 4–6 weeks if symptoms persist or return. Partial relief of symptoms is an indication for a repeat injection. A total of three injections in a given 12-month period is the accepted standard (hyaluronic acid is given as a series of three to five weekly injections and can be repeated in 6 months). If significant pain relief is not obtained after three injections, consider further imaging studies and possible surgical consultation.

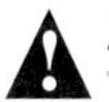

Acromioclavicular Joint

Name of Procedure

Intraarticular injection of the acromioclavicular joint is the name of the procedure.

CPT

The Current Procedural Terminology code is 20605 (injection of intermediate joint).

Indications

Intraarticular injections of the acromioclavicular (AC) joint are usually performed for pain secondary to arthritis (most commonly posttraumatic arthritis) or for grade 1 AC ligament sprains. Injections that use only local anesthetic (rather than an anesthetic and corticosteroid mixture) can be done for diagnostic purposes. This will help differentiate the source of pain as the AC joint (rather than other structures such as joints, tendons, or bursa.) Relief of pain after a local anesthetic injection into the AC joint indicates that the AC joint is the pain generator.

Symptoms

- Pain localized and stiffness localized to the acromioclavicular joint.
- Pain worse with reaching across the chest or behind the back.
- Patient may be unable to sleep on the affected shoulder.

Physical Examination Findings

- May see swelling of the joint with tenderness to palpation.

Medications to Inject

A corticosteroid and local anesthetic mixture is injected.

Amount to Inject

The injection should be 1–1½ cc.

Size and Gauge of Needle

A ⅝–1-inch 25-gauge needle is used.

Local Anatomy

The acromioclavicular joint articulates the distal end of the clavicle with the anterior, medial aspect of the acromion. Dense ligaments strengthen and stabilize the joint.

Patient Position

The patient should be comfortably seated with the hand of the affected shoulder placed on the lap.

How and Where to Inject

Standing behind the patient, palpate the sulcus formed by the distal end of the clavicle and its articulation with the dorsomedial surface of the acromion. Inject in this location just medial to the acromion. If the needle hits the bone, the needle is withdrawn slightly and redirected into the joint space. The needle may not pass deeply into the joint space. There should be little resistance to injection if the needle is in the joint, although only a small volume will be able to be injected. If there is resistance, the needle may be in

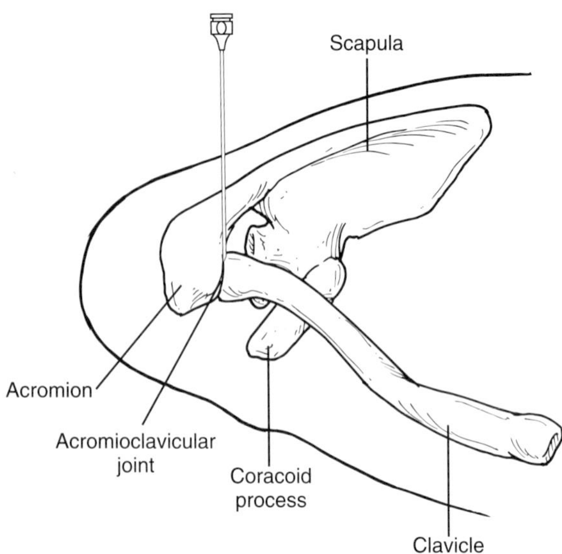

Fig 3–5 Acromioclavicular joint injection.

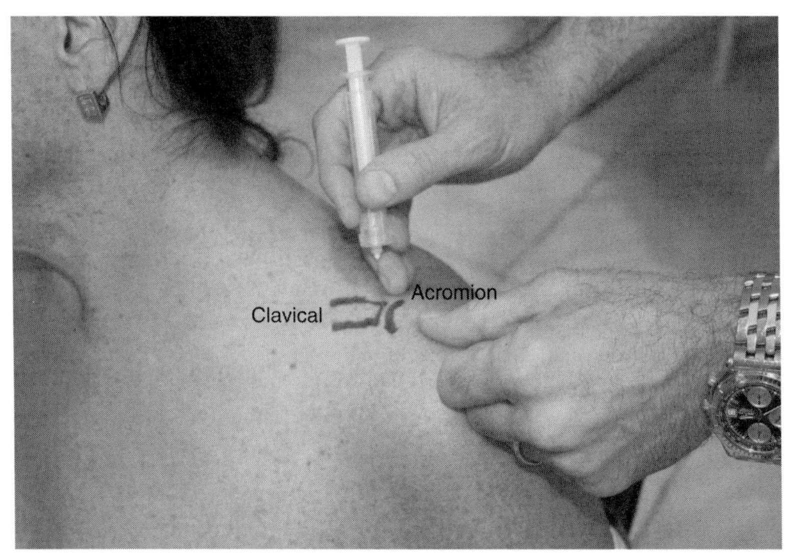

Fig 3–6 Acromioclavicular joint injection.

a ligament, and the position should be changed. Aspirate the joint before injecting to avoid intravascular administration (Figures 3–5 and 3–6).

Pitfalls/Complications

X-rays should be taken of the joint before injection. Do not inject the joint if acute infection is suspected. It is anticipated that the patient may have an increase in pain for a few days caused by the use of corticosteroids. Informing patients of this helps to alleviate their postinjection pain concerns. If there is no relief from the injection, consider the possibility of a missed injection (outside the joint), as well as other sources of pain (fractures, rotator cuff tear, rotator cuff tendinitis, infection, joint instability caused by ligamentous disruption, bursitis). The chance of infection can be minimized by Betadine preparation and aseptic technique. Bursitis and/or tendinitis may coexist and may require additional treatment.

Postinjection Care

Apply a sterile dressing and pressure over the injection site. Have the patient ice the affected area for 20 minutes two to three times daily for the first 24–48 hours. Then begin local heat and gentle stretching exercises several days after the injection. Avoid vigorous exercise, lifting, or overhead activities for several days.

When to Perform Follow-Up Injections

Although there are no strict guidelines, a reasonable approach is to reinject in 4–6 weeks if symptoms persist or return. Partial relief of symptoms is an indication for a repeat injection. A total of three injections in a given 12-month period is the accepted standard. If significant pain relief is not obtained after three injections, consider further imaging studies and possible surgical consultation.

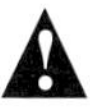

Sternoclavicular Joint

Name of Procedure

Intraarticular injection of the sternoclavicular joint is the name of this procedure.

CPT

The Current Procedural Terminology code is 20600 (injection of small joint).

Indications

Intraarticular injections of the sternoclavicular joint are usually performed for pain secondary to arthritis (most commonly osteoarthritis, rheumatoid arthritis, ankylosing spondylitis, Reiter's syndrome, or psoriatic arthritis). Injection is usually offered after a patient has had a course of NSAID and/or physical therapy fail.

Symptoms

- Pain localized to the sternum. Patient may feel he/she is experiencing a myocardial infarction.
- Pain worse with activity of the shoulder.

Physical Examination Findings

- Pain reproduced with active protraction or retraction of the shoulder or arm elevation.
- Joint may be tender to palpation.
- Clicking may be noted on range of motion.
- Patient may splint the joint by keeping the shoulders in neutral.

Medications to Inject

A corticosteroid and local anesthetic mixture is injected.

Amount to Inject

The injection amount is 1mL.

Size and Gauge of Needle

A 1–1½-inch 25-gauge needle is used. The length of the needle will depend on how much subcutaneous tissue is in the affected area. People who have more adipose tissue will require the use of a longer needle.

Local Anatomy

The sternoclavicular joint is a true joint with synovial lining. It is the articulation of the sternal end of the clavicle, the sternal manubrium, and the cartilage of the first rib. On the left side, the common carotid artery and the brachiocephalic vein runs posterior to the joint. On the right side, the brachiocephalic artery is posterior to the joint. These vessels are susceptible to injury if the injection is performed too deeply. Ligaments surround the joints and help to strengthen them.

Patient Position

The patient is placed in the supine position.

How and Where to Inject

The sternal end of the clavicle is palpated. The sternoclavicular joint is noted as the indentation where the clavicle meets the sternal manubrium. The needle is inserted at the middle of this indentation and advanced medially at a 45-degree angle into the joint. If the needle hits the bone, the needle is withdrawn slightly and redirected into the joint space (Figures 3–7 and 3–8). This is a relatively superficial injection, and the needle should be advanced only slightly past the ligament because the brachiocephalic vessels are located beneath. There should be some resistance to injection if the needle is in the joint because the joint space is small. If there is significant resistance, the needle may be in a ligament, and the position should be changed. Aspirate before injecting to avoid intravascular administration.

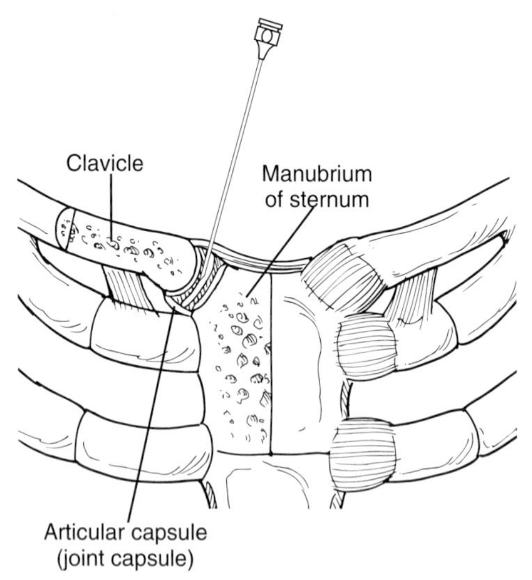

Fig 3–7 Sternoclavicular joint injection.

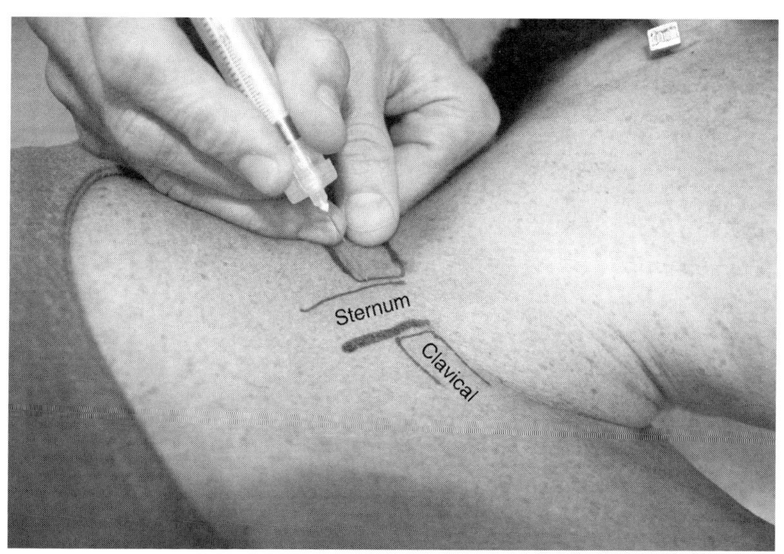

Fig 3–8 Sternoclavicular joint injection.

Pitfalls/Complications

Because inflammation of this joint is sometimes confused with myocardial infarction, cardiac disease should be ruled out. X-rays should be taken of the joint before injection. Do not inject too deeply because veins, arteries, and the lung lie posteriorly. Always aspirate before injecting. It is anticipated that the patient may have an increase in pain for a few days because of the use of corticosteroids. Informing patients of this helps to alleviate their postinjection pain concerns. If there is no relief from the injection, consider other sources of pain (fractures, tumor, bursitis, tendinitis, infection). The use of Betadine preparation and sterile technique can minimize the risk of infection.

Postinjection Care

Apply a sterile dressing and pressure over the injection site. Have the patient ice the affected area for 20 minutes two to three times daily for the first 24–48 hours. Then begin local heat and gentle stretching exercises several days after the injection. Avoid vigorous exercise, sleeping on the affected side, or overhead activity for several days.

When to Perform Follow-Up Injections

Although there are no strict guidelines, a reasonable approach is to reinject in 4–6 weeks if symptoms persist or return. Partial relief of symptoms is an indication for a repeat injection. A total of three injections in a given 12-month period is the accepted standard. If significant pain relief is not obtained after three injections, consider further imaging studies.

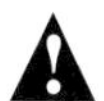

Elbow Joint

Name of Procedure

Intraarticular injection of the elbow joint is the name of the procedure.

CPT

The Current Procedural Terminology code is 20605 (injection of intermediate joint).

Indications

Intraarticular injections of the elbow are usually performed for pain secondary to arthritis (most commonly rheumatoid arthritis or traumatic osteoarthritis). Injection is usually offered after a patient has had a course of NSAID and/or physical therapy fail.

Symptoms

- Pain and stiffness localized to the elbow (in any joint disease, pain may radiate to the joint above and the joint below).
- Pain worse with activity.
- Decreased functional status secondary to pain and decreased range of motion.
- Associated ulnar neuropathy at the elbow may be present with tingling in the fourth and fifth digits.

Physical Examination Findings

- Decreased passive range of motion of the joint, usually in extension.
- Crepitus may be noted on range of motion.
- Joint flexion contracture or elbow instability may be present.
- Tinel's sign at the medial elbow (ulnar groove) and decreased sensation in the fourth and fifth digits may indicate associated ulnar neuropathy at the elbow.

Medications to Inject

A corticosteroid and local anesthetic mixture is injected. Some physicians prefer injecting hyaluronic acid.

Amounto Inject

The amount of the injection is 4–6 cc.

Size and Gauge of Needle

A 1–1½-inch 23-gauge needle is used. The length of the needle will depend on how much subcutaneous tissue is in the affected area.

Local Anatomy

The elbow joint is formed by the articulation of the humerus, radius, and ulna. The ulnar collateral ligament lies medially, and the radial collateral ligament lies laterally. The olecranon bursa lies posterior to the elbow joint. Bursae are also located between the insertion of the biceps and the head of the radius, as well as the cubital and antecubital areas.

Patient Position

The patient should be seated or supine with the elbow flexed 50–90 degrees.

How and Where to Inject

For a posterior lateral approach, the needle is inserted in the center of a triangle formed by the lateral epicondyle, the radial head, and the tip of the olecranon (Figures 3–9 and 3–10). The lateral epicondyle and the posterior olecranon are palpated. Inject proximally

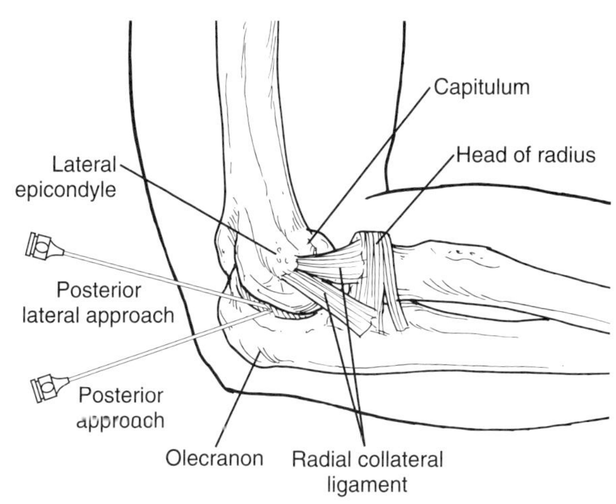

Fig 3–9 Elbow joint injection.

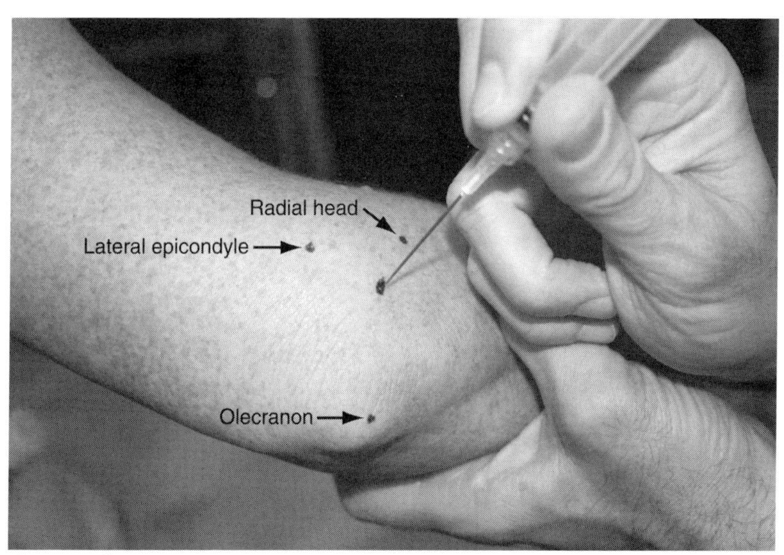

Fig 3–10 Elbow joint injection.

toward the head of the radius and medially into the joint. The posterior approach may also be used. The needle is inserted above the superior lateral aspect of the olecranon. If the needle hits the bone, the needle is withdrawn slightly and redirected into the joint space. There should be little resistance to injection if the needle is in the joint. If there is resistance, the needle may be in a ligament or tendon, and the position should be changed. Aspirate the joint before injecting to avoid intravascular administration. Avoid injecting if aspirate appears infected. Do not inject corticosteroids if there is any suspicion that the joint is infected.

Pitfalls/Complications

X-rays should be taken of the joint before injection. Use a posterolateral or posterior approach to avoid nerves and blood vessels. A posterolateral approach avoids the vessels and nerves in the cubital and antecubital spaces. Note the radial nerve crosses the elbow joint medial to the brachioradialis; if the injection is too medial, it can be in the vicinity of this nerve. It is anticipated that the patient may have an increase in pain for a few days caused by the use of corticosteroids. Informing patients of this helps to alleviate their postinjection pain concerns. If there is no relief from the injection, consider other sources of pain (fractures, bursitis, tendinitis, nerve entrapments, gout, pseudogout, seronegative spondyloarthropathies, systemic lupus erythematosus, medial or lateral epicondylitis, cubital tunnel syndrome, elbow contracture, infection). The use of Betadine preparation and sterile technique can minimize the risk of infection. Bursitis and/or tendinitis may coexist and may require additional treatment.

Postinjection Care

Apply a sterile dressing and pressure over the injection site. Have the patient ice the affected area for 20 minutes two to three times daily for the first 24–48 hours. A sling may be used for relative rest of the joint. Remove the elbow from the sling several times a day for range of motion exercises. Then begin local heat and gentle stretching exercises several days after the injection. Avoid vigorous exercise for several days.

When to Perform Follow-Up Injections

Although there are no strict guidelines, a reasonable approach is to reinject in 4–6 weeks if symptoms persist or return. Partial relief of symptoms is an indication for a repeat injection. A total of three injections in a given 12-month period is the accepted standard (hyaluronic acid is given as a series of three to five weekly injections and can be repeated in 6 months). If significant pain relief is not obtained after three injections, consider further imaging studies and possible surgical consultation.

Wrist Joint

Name of Procedure

Intraarticular injection of the wrist joint is the name of the procedure.

CPT

The Current Procedural Terminology code is 20605 (injection of intermediate joint).

Indications

Intraarticular injections of the wrist joint are usually performed for pain secondary to arthritis (most commonly after scapholunate advance collapse or triscaphe arthritis). Pain may also be due to primary osteoarthritis or rheumatoid arthritis. Injection is usually offered after a patient has had a course of splinting of the wrist (in a neutral position) and NSAID therapy fail.

Symptoms

- Pain and stiffness localized to the wrist joint, usually on the radial side (in any joint disease, pain may radiate to the joint above and the joint below).
- Pain worse with activity.

- Decreased functional status in pinch or grip strength secondary to pain and decreased range of motion.

Physical Examination Findings

- Decreased passive range of motion of the joint (pain more likely at the extreme ranges of motion than throughout the entire range).
- Decreased pinch strength.
- Crepitus may be noted on range of motion.

Medications to Inject

A corticosteroid and local anesthetic mixture (do not use anesthetic with epinephrine) is used.

Amount to Inject

The injection amount is 1–2 cc.

Size and Gauge of Needle

A ¾-inch 25-gauge needle is used.

Local Anatomy

The wrist joint generally refers to the radiocarpal joint, which is the articulation between the distal end of the radius and the articulating surface of the scaphoid, lunate, and triquetral bones. Other articulations in the wrist area include the distal radius and ulnar and the carpal bones. Medial, lateral, anterior, and posterior ligaments strengthen the joint. Anteriorly, the flexor tendons bind the wrist, and the median and ulnar nerves are in close proximity to these tendons. The extensor tendons are located posteriorly. The radial artery runs laterally, and the dorsal branch of the ulnar nerve runs medially. Because many of the joints of the wrist have interconnecting synovial spaces, relief in the wrist may be obtained by one injection.

Patient Position

The hand should be resting comfortably on the table with the wrist slightly elevated on a towel with the wrist pronated.

How and Where to Inject

The radial carpal joint can be palpated on the dorsum of the wrist, just distal to the distal edge of the radius. Locate the extensor indicis and extensor pollicis longus tendons as they pass distal to the radius. The needle can be inserted just distal to the radius (Figures 3–11 and 3–12).

The wrist can also be injected with an ulnar approach. The needle can be injected just distal to the lateral ulna between the distal ulna and the carpal bones. If the needle hits the bone, the needle is withdrawn slightly into the joint space. There should be little resistance to injection if the needle is in the joint. If there is resistance, the needle may be in a ligament or tendon, and the position should be changed. Aspirate the joint before injecting to avoid intravascular administration. Avoid injecting if aspirate appears infected.

Pitfalls/Complications

X-rays should be taken of the joint before injection. Do not inject the joint if acute infection is suspected. It is anticipated that the patient may have an increase in pain for a few

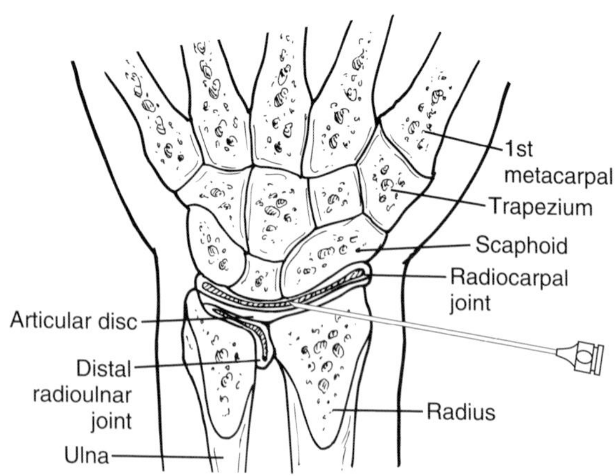

Fig 3–11 Wrist joint (radial carpal) injection.

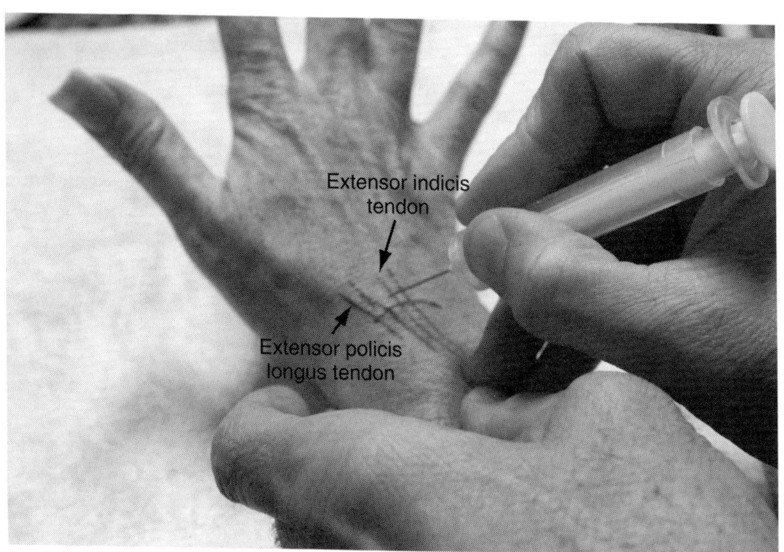

Fig 3–12 Wrist joint (radial carpal) injection.

days caused by the use of corticosteroids. Informing patients of this helps to alleviate their postinjection pain concerns. If there is no relief from the injection, consider other sources of pain (fractures, gout, pseudogout, scapholunate dislocation, carpal instability, tendinitis, avascular necrosis, infection). The use of Betadine preparation and sterile technique can minimize the risk of infection. Tendinitis may coexist and may require additional treatment.

Postinjection Care

Apply a sterile dressing and pressure over the injection site. Range of motion exercises after the injection may help the medications infuse throughout the joint. Have the patient ice the affected area for 20 minutes two to three times daily for the first 24–48 hours. Some physicians advocate splinting the wrist for 1 day after the injection. Begin local heat and gentle stretching exercises several days after the injection.

When to Perform Follow-Up Injections

Although there are no strict guidelines, a reasonable approach is to reinject in 4–6 weeks if symptoms persist or return. Partial relief of symptoms is an indication for a repeat injection. A total of three injections in a given 12-month period is the accepted standard. If significant pain relief is not obtained after three injections, consider further imaging studies and possible surgical consultation. Surgical treatment may be necessary if hand function is affected.

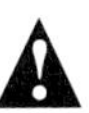

Intercarpal Joint

Name of Procedure

Intraarticular injection of the intercarpal joints is the name of the procedure.

CPT

The Current Procedural Terminology code is 20605 (injection of intermediate joint).

Indications

Intraarticular injections of the intercarpal joint are usually performed for pain secondary to arthritis (most commonly osteoarthritis or rheumatoid arthritis). Injection is usually offered after a patient has a course of NSAID and/or physical therapy fail.

Symptoms

- Pain and stiffness localized to the intercarpal joint (in any joint disease, pain may radiate to the joint above and the joint below).
- Pain worse with wrist activity.

Physical Examination Findings

- Decreased passive range of motion of the wrist.
- Crepitus may be noted on range of motion.

Medications to Inject

A corticosteroid and local anesthetic mixture (do not use anesthetic with epinephrine) is injected. Some physicians prefer injecting hyaluronic acid.

Amount to Inject

The injectate amount is 1–2 mL.

Size and Gauge of Needle

A 1-inch 25-gauge needle is used.

Local Anatomy

The eight carpal bones articulate with each other, the metacarpals, the radius, and the ulna.

Patient Position

The patient is positioned with the palm down and the hand resting comfortably on a towel.

How and Where to Inject

The intercarpal joint can be injected by palpating the borders of the affected carpal bone. Some physicians prefer to do the injection under fluoroscopic guidance for precise location. If the needle hits the bone, the needle is withdrawn slightly and redirected into the joint space. There should be little resistance to injection if the needle is in the joint. If there is resistance, the needle may be in a ligament or tendon, and the position should be changed. Aspirate the joint before injecting to ensure that infection is not present and to avoid intravascular administration (Figures 3–13 and 3–14).

Pitfalls/Complications

X-rays should be taken of the joint before injection. Do not inject the joint if acute infection is suspected. It is anticipated that the patient may have an increase in pain for a few days caused by the use of corticosteroids. Informing patients of this helps to alleviate their postinjection pain concerns. If there is no relief from the injection, consider other sources of pain (fractures, tendinitis, infection). The risk of infection can be minimized with sterile preparation of the area and aseptic technique. Tendinitis may coexist and may require additional treatment.

Postinjection Care

Apply a sterile dressing and pressure over the injection site. Have the patient ice the affected area for 20 minutes two to three times daily for the first 24–48 hours. Then begin

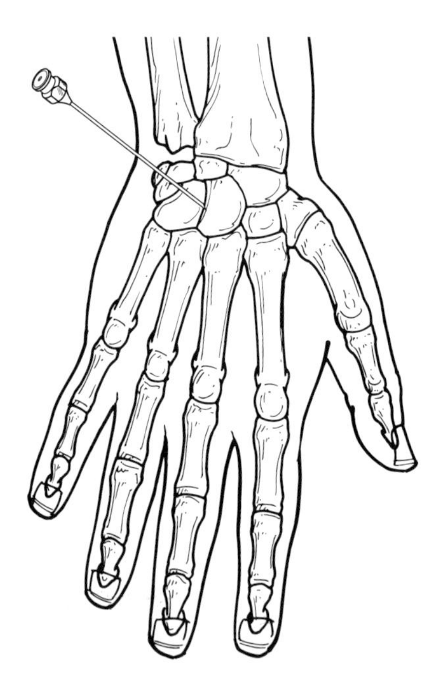

Fig 3–13 Intercarpal joint injection.

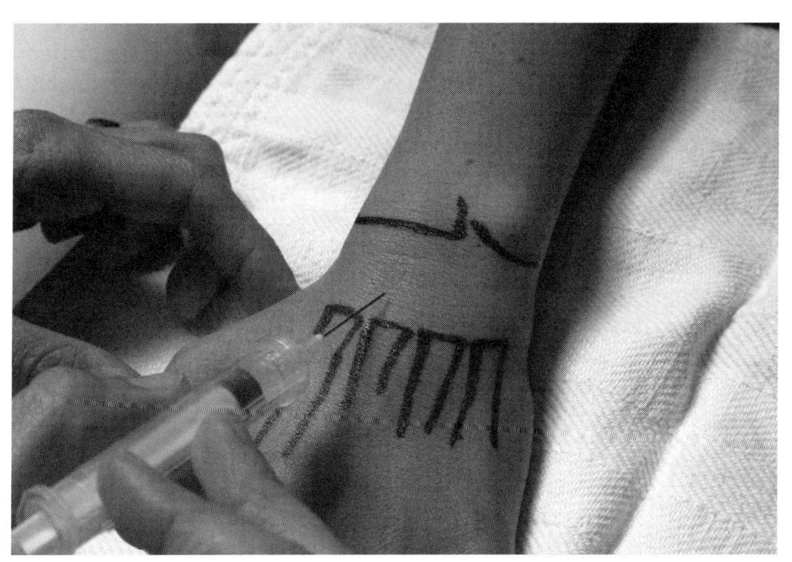

Fig 3–14 Intercarpal joint injection.

local heat and gentle stretching exercises several days after the injection. Avoid vigorous exercise or use of the wrist for several days.

When to Perform Follow-Up Injections

Although there are no strict guidelines, a reasonable approach is to reinject in 4–6 weeks if symptoms persist or return. Partial relief of symptoms is an indication for a repeat injection. A total of three injections in a given 12-month period is the accepted standard (hyaluronic acid is given as a series of three to five weekly injections and can be repeated in 6 months). If significant pain relief is not obtained after three injections, consider further imaging studies and possible surgical consultation.

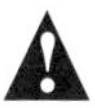

First Carpometacarpal Joint

Name of Procedure

Intraarticular injection of the first carpometacarpal joint is the name of this procedure.

CPT

The Current Procedural Terminology code is 20600 (injection of small joint).

Indications

Intraarticular injections of the first metacarpal joints are usually performed for pain secondary to arthritis (most commonly osteoarthritis or rheumatoid arthritis). Injection is usually offered after a patient has had a course of splinting (thumb spica splint) and NSAID therapy fail.

Symptoms

- Pain and stiffness localized to the first carpometacarpal joint (in any joint disease, pain may radiate to the joint above and the joint below).

- Pain worse with activity.
- Decreased functional status in pinch and grip strength secondary to pain and decreased range of motion.

Physical Examination Findings

- Decreased passive range of motion of the joint.
- Decreased pinch strength.
- Positive Watson's stress test (with the palm up and the MP and IP joints extended, the thumb is pushed down, resulting in pain).
- Crepitus may be noted on range of motion.
- Flexion contracture of the thumb may be noted.

Medications to Inject

A corticosteroid and local anesthetic mixture (do not use anesthetic with epinephrine) is used.

Amount to Inject

The injectate amount is 1–2.5 cc.

Size and Gauge of Needle

A ¾-inch 25- or 27-gauge needle is used.

Local Anatomy

The first carpometacarpal joint lies between the trapezium and the base of the first metacarpal.

Patient Position

The hand should be resting comfortably on the table in a neutral position between supination and pronation (radial side up), with the wrist slightly elevated on a towel.

How and Where to Inject

Inject the first carpometacarpal joint from the volar radial side of the thumb. To locate the joint space, gently pull upward on the thumb and palpate the base of the metacarpal. The examiner should palpate the proximal metacarpal and slide his/her finger proximally until a "step-off" is felt. This is the carpometacarpal joint. Inject adjacent to the abductor pollicis longus tendon (Figures 3–15 and 3–16). If the needle hits the bone (trapezium), the needle is withdrawn slightly and redirected into the joint space. There should be little resistance to injection if the needle is in the joint. If there is resistance, the needle may be in a ligament or tendon, and the position should be changed. Avoid the radial artery, and be sure to aspirate before injecting to make sure you are not in the artery.

Pitfalls/Complications

X-rays should be taken of the joint before injection. Do not inject the joint if acute infection is suspected. It is anticipated that the patient may have an increase in pain for a few days caused by the use of corticosteroids. Informing patients of this helps to alleviate their postinjection pain concerns. Avoid the radial artery. The radial sensory nerve is in the area of this injection, and the patient should be cautioned to alert the examiner if

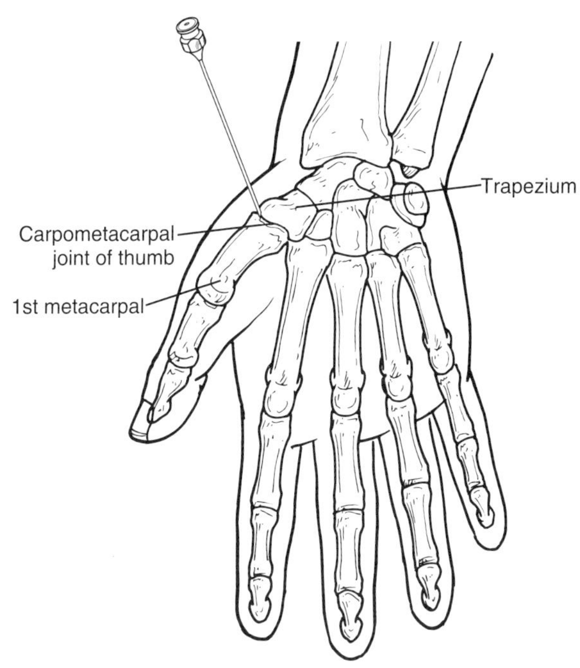

Fig 3–15 First carpometacarpal joint injection.

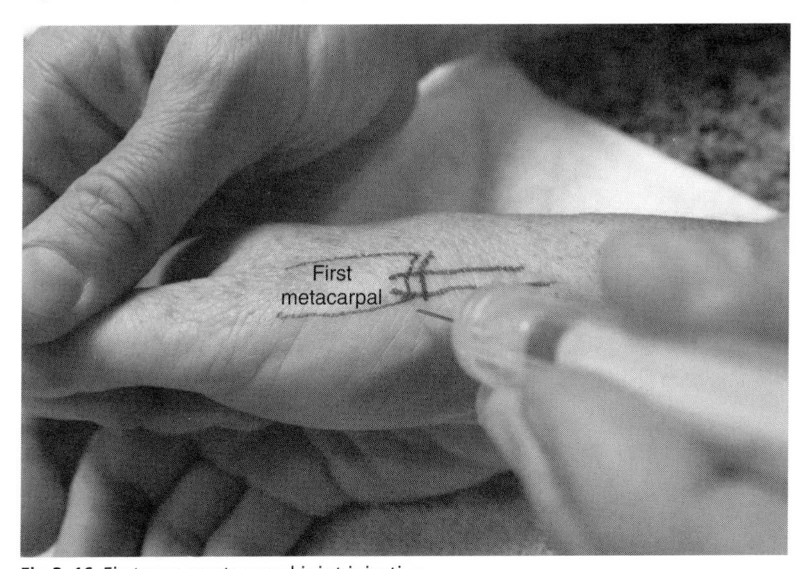

Fig 3–16 First carpometacarpal joint injection.

paresthesias occur during injection. The patient should be aware that this nerve might be injured during this injection. The abductor pollicis longus and extensor pollicis longus and brevis are also in this area, and these can be injured during injection. Care should be used to avoid intraneural or intratendinous injections. Aspirating before injecting will ensure that you are not in the artery. If there is no relief from the injection, consider other sources of pain (fractures of the scaphoid or other carpal bones including the trapezium, carpal tunnel syndrome, de Quervain's tenosynovitis, tendinitis, infection). The use of Betadine preparation and sterile technique can minimize the risk of infection. Tendinitis may coexist and may require additional treatment.

Postinjection Care

Apply a sterile dressing and pressure over the injection site. Have the patient ice the affected area for 20 minutes two to three times daily for the first 24–48 hours. Local heat and gentle thumb stretching exercises in flexion and extension can be started several days after the injection. Apply a thumb spica splint for the first 3 days after the injection.

When to Perform Follow-Up Injections

Although there are no strict guidelines, a reasonable approach is to reinject in 4–6 weeks if symptoms persist or return. Partial relief of symptoms is an indication for a repeat injection. A total of three injections in a given 12-month period is the accepted standard. If significant pain relief is not obtained after three injections, consider further imaging studies and possible surgical consultation.

Interphalangeal Joints

Name of Procedure

Intraarticular injection of the interphalangeal joints is the name of this procedure.

CPT

The Current Procedural Terminology code is 20600 (injection of small joint).

Indications

Intraarticular injections of the interphalangeal joints are usually performed for pain secondary to arthritis (most commonly osteoarthritis or rheumatoid arthritis). Injection is usually offered after a patient has had a course of splinting and NSAID therapy fail.

Symptoms

- Pain and stiffness localized to the interphalangeal joint.
- Pain worse with activity.
- Decreased functional status in pinch and grip strength secondary to pain and decreased range of motion.

Physical Examination Findings

- Decreased passive range of motion of the interphalangeal joint.
- Decreased pinch strength.
- Heberden (distal interphalangeal joint) or Bouchard's (proximal interphalangeal joint) nodes may be present.
- Crepitus may be noted on range of motion.
- Flexion contracture of the thumb may be noted.

Medications to Inject

A corticosteroid and local anesthetic mixture (do not use anesthetic with epinephrine) is injected.

Amount to Inject

The injectate amount is 0.5–1 cc.

Size and Gauge of Needle

A ¾–1-inch 25- or 27-gauge needle is used.

Local Anatomy

The interphalangeal joints lie between the proximal and middle phalanges (proximal interphalangeal joint or PIP) and middle and distal phalanges (distal interphalangeal joint or DIP) in each of the fingers (except in the thumb, which has only proximal and distal phalanges and one interphalangeal joint). Ligaments surround the joints and help to strengthen them.

Patient Position

The hand should be resting comfortably on the table with the palm down. The wrist can be slightly elevated on a towel.

How and Where to Inject

Identify the joint by flexing and extending the joint. After marking the skin and sterile prep, vapocoolant spray should be used to provide topical anesthesia. Insert the needle on the dorsum of the digit in the center of the joint space (Figures 3–17 and 3–18). This approach avoids the digital nerves, which are on the radial and ulnar side of the digits. If the needle hits the bone, the needle is withdrawn slightly and redirected into the joint space. Applying traction to the digit may open the joint space and ease injection. There should be little resistance to injection if the needle is in the joint, although because the joint is very small, resistance will increase after 0.5–1 mL is injected. If there is resistance, the needle may be in a ligament or tendon, and the position should be changed. Aspirate before injecting to avoid intravascular administration.

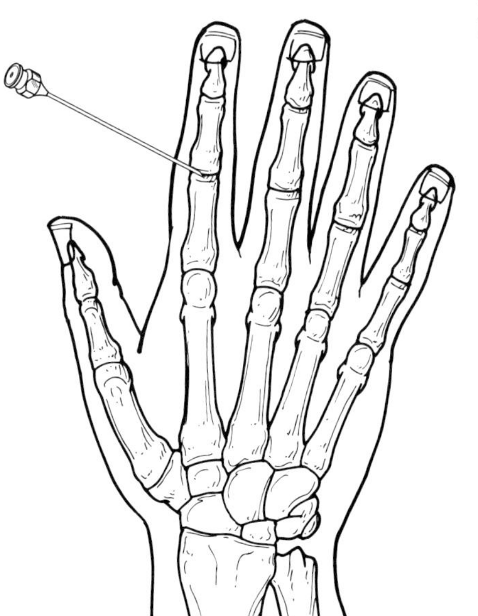

Fig 3–17 Interphalangeal joint injection.

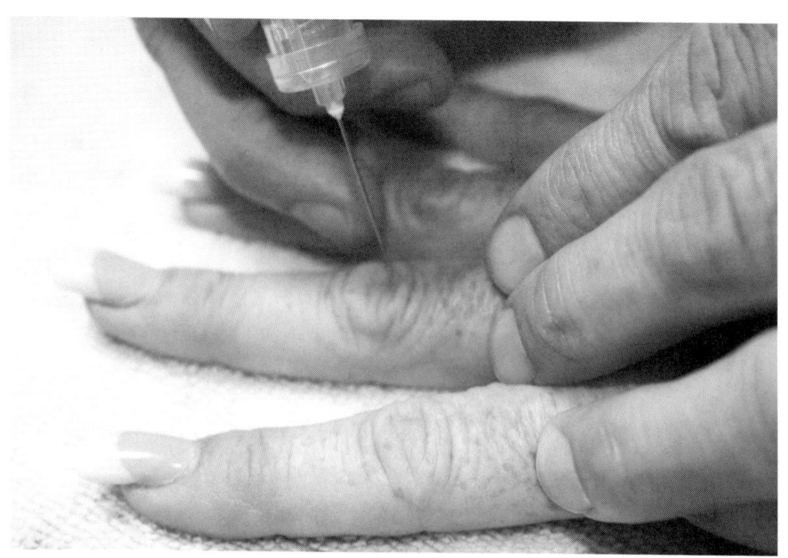

Fig 3–18 Interphalangeal joint injection.

Pitfalls/Complications

X-rays should be taken of the joint before injection. Do not inject the joint if acute infection is suspected. It is anticipated that the patient may have an increase in pain for a few days caused by the use of corticosteroids. Informing patients of this helps to alleviate their postinjection pain concerns. If there is no relief from the injection, consider other sources of pain (fractures, tendinitis, infection). The risk of infection can be minimized with sterile preparation of the area and aseptic technique. Tendinitis may coexist and may require additional treatment.

Postinjection Care

Apply a sterile dressing and pressure over the injection site. Have the patient ice the affected area for 20 minutes two to three times daily for the first 24–48 hours. Then begin local heat and gentle stretching exercises several days after the injection.

When to Perform Follow-Up Injections

Although there are no strict guidelines, a reasonable approach is to reinject in 4–6 weeks if symptoms persist or return. Partial relief of symptoms is an indication for a repeat injection. A total of three injections in a given 12-month period is the accepted standard. If significant pain relief is not obtained after three injections, consider further imaging studies and possible surgical consultation.

Temporomandibular Joint

Name of Procedure

Intraarticular injection of the temporomandibular joint is the name of this procedure.

CPT

The Current Procedural Terminology code is 20605 (injection of intermediate joint).

Indications

Intraarticular injections of the temporomandibular joint are usually performed for pain secondary to temporomandibular joint syndrome (chronic irritation of the joint secondary to grinding of the teeth or malocclusion), posttraumatic arthritis, or rheumatoid arthritis. Injection is usually offered after a patient has had a course of muscle relaxants, NSAIDs, low-dose tricyclic antidepressant medication, use of an orthotic, or soft diet fails.

Symptoms

- Pain and stiffness localized to the temporomandibular joint. The pain can radiate to the ear, neck, mandible, and tonsils.
- Patient may complain of popping, clicking, grinding, or crepitation.
- Stress can aggravate the condition.
- Headache is common.

Physical Examination Findings

- Decreased jaw opening may be noted.
- With a finger over the temporomandibular joint, clicking or grating of the joint may be noted when the patient opens and closes the mouth.
- Dental malocclusion may be noted.

Medications to Inject

A corticosteroid and local anesthetic mixture is used.

Amount to Inject

The injectate amount is 0.5–1 mL.

Size and Gauge of Needle

A 1-inch 25- to 27-gauge needle is used.

Local Anatomy

The temporomandibular joint is a hinge joint that lies between the mandible and the temporal bone. A fibrous articular disc lies between the bones. Ligaments, the muscles of mastication, and the joint capsule support it. The temporal artery runs nearby.

Patient Position

The patient is placed in the supine position with the head facing away (side being injected up).

How and Where to Inject

The injection may be done with the mouth open or closed. With the mouth open, the needle is inserted approximately ½ inch anterior to the tragus. With the mouth closed and the teeth not clenched, the zygomatic arch (adjacent to the condylar process of the mandible) is palpated. Insert the needle ½ inch inferiorly. A pop will be felt when the joint is entered. Aspirate before injecting to avoid intravascular injection (the temporal artery runs posterior to this joint). If the needle hits the bone, the needle is withdrawn slightly and redirected into the joint space. There should be little resistance to injection if the needle is in the joint. If there is resistance, the needle may be in a ligament or tendon, and the position should be changed (Figures 3–19 and 3–20). Some physicians prefer to aspirate the joint before injecting to ensure that infection or hemarthrosis is not present.

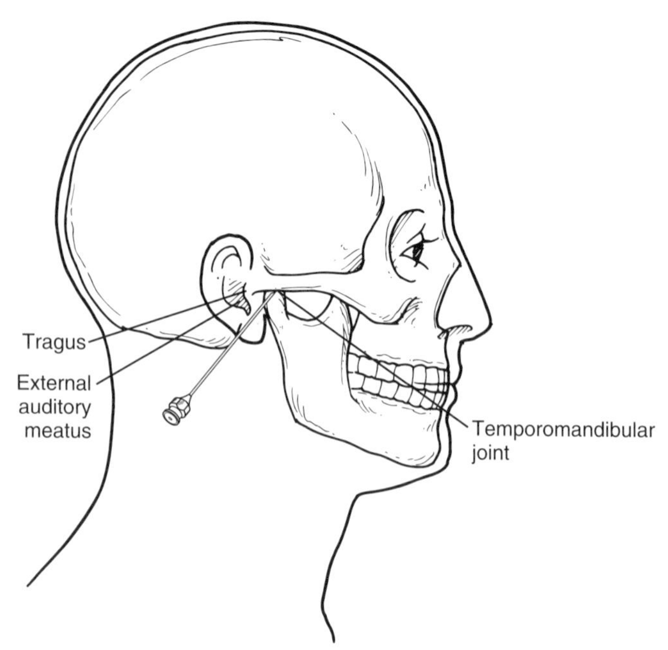

Fig 3–19 Temporomandibular joint injection.

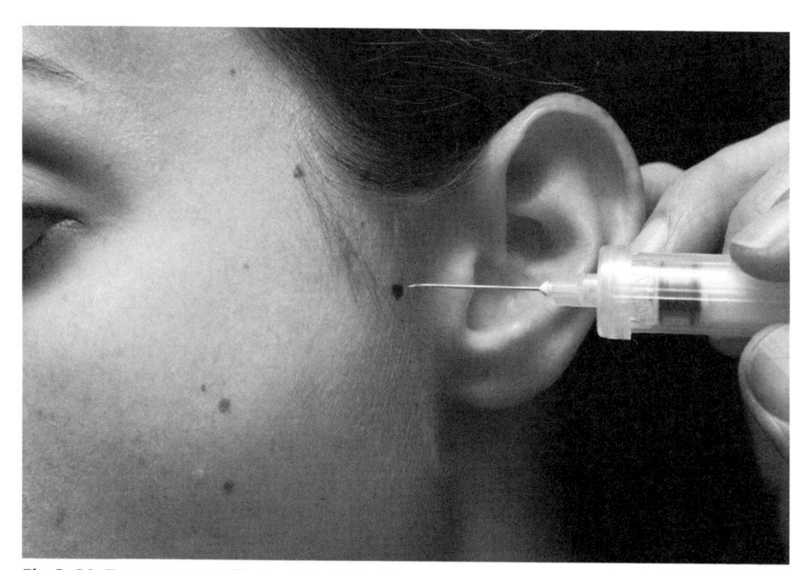

Fig 3–20 Temporomandibular joint injection.

Pitfalls/Complications

The temporal artery courses posteriorly and should be avoided. Aspirate before injecting to ensure that the needle is not in a blood vessel. Ecchymosis and hematomas may be evident after the injection, and the patient should be warned of this. Blockade of the facial nerve is a complication, with associated facial muscle weakness. X-rays should be taken of the joint before injection. Do not inject the joint if acute infection is suspected. It is anticipated that the patient may have an increase in pain for a few days caused by the use of corticosteroids. Informing patients of this helps to alleviate their postinjection pain concerns. If there is no relief from the injection, consider other sources of pain (fractures, tumor, infection, facial nerve injuries, headaches, collagen vascular disease, jaw claudication associated with temporal arteritis). The risk of infection can be minimized with sterile preparation of the area and aseptic technique. Myofascial pain may coexist and may require additional treatment. Occasionally, use of a dental orthotic or trigger point injections may be helpful.

Postinjection Care

Apply a sterile dressing and pressure over the injection site. Have the patient ice the affected area for 20 minutes two to three times daily for the first 24–48 hours.

When to Perform Follow-Up Injections

Although there are no strict guidelines, a reasonable approach is to reinject in 4–6 weeks if symptoms persist or return. Partial relief of symptoms is an indication for a repeat injection. A total of three injections in a given 12-month period is the accepted standard. If significant pain relief is not obtained after three injections, consider referral to an oral surgeon.

Hip Joint

Name of Procedure

Intraarticular injection of the hip joint is the name of this procedure.

CPT

The Current Procedural Terminology code is 20610 (injection of major joint).

Indications

Intraarticular injections of the hip are usually performed for pain secondary to arthritis (most commonly osteoarthritis or rheumatoid arthritis). Injection is usually offered after a patient has had a course of NSAID, assistive devices such as canes, weight loss, and/or physical therapy fail and before joint replacement is considered.

Symptoms

- Pain and stiffness localized to the hip and upper leg (in any joint disease, pain may radiate to the joint above and the joint below).
- Pain worse with activity.
- Hip joint stiffness after inactivity.
- Decreased functional status in ambulation secondary to pain and decreased range of motion.

Physical Examination Findings

- Decreased passive range of motion of the hip joint.
- Crepitus may be noted on range of motion.
- Antalgic gait.

Medications to Inject

A corticosteroid and local anesthetic mixture is injected. Some physicians prefer injecting hyaluronic acid.

Amount to Inject

The injectate amount is 5 mL.

Size and Gauge of Needle

A 2-inch 25-gauge needle is used. The length of the needle will depend on how much subcutaneous tissue is in the affected area. People who have more adipose tissue will require the use of a longer needle.

Local Anatomy

The head of the femur articulates with the acetabulum of the hip.

Patient Position

The patient is placed in the supine position for an anterior approach. The patient is placed in a side lying position on the unaffected side for a lateral approach.

How and Where to Inject

Some physicians recommend fluoroscopic guidance for accurate needle placement.

Anterior Approach

The femoral artery is palpated and marked. The hip joint is located approximately 2 inches lateral to the femoral artery just below the inguinal ligament. This site is marked. After Betadine preparation and under aseptic conditions, the needle is inserted at this site. Advance the needle through the skin and subcutaneous tissues through the joint capsule and into the joint. If the needle hits the bone, the needle is withdrawn slightly and redirected into the joint space. There should be little resistance to injection if the needle is in the joint. If there is resistance, the needle may be in a ligament or tendon, and the position should be changed. Aspirate the joint before injecting to avoid intravascular administration. If aspirate appears infected, discontinue the injection (Figures 3–21 and 3–22).

Lateral Approach

With the patient lying on the pain-free side, palpate and mark the greater trochanter. After Betadine preparation and using aseptic technique, insert the needle 1–2 cm proximal to the greater trochanter. Advance the needle through the skin and subcutaneous tissues through the joint capsule and into the joint. If the needle hits the bone, the needle is withdrawn slightly and redirected into the joint space. There should be little resistance to injection if the needle is in the joint. If there is resistance, the needle may be in a ligament or tendon, and the position should be changed. Aspirate the joint before injecting to avoid intravascular administration. If aspirate appears infected, discontinue injection (Figures 3–23 and 3–24).

Pitfalls/Complications

X-rays should be taken of the hip before injection. Do not inject the joint if acute infection is suspected. It is anticipated that the patient may have an increase in pain for a few days caused by the use of corticosteroids. Informing patients of this helps to alleviate

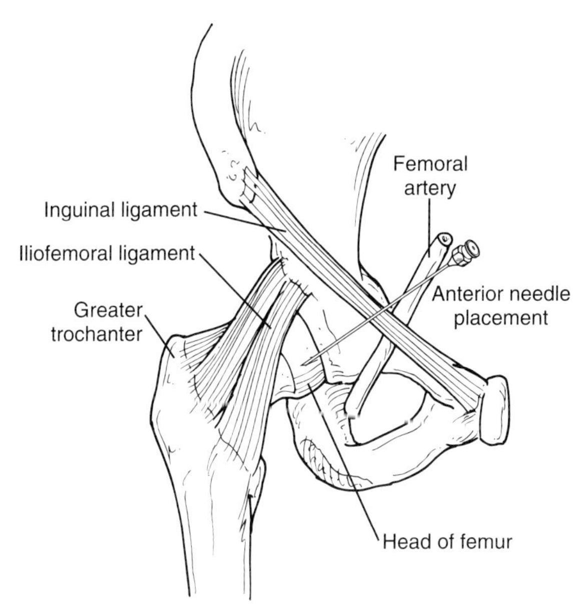

Fig 3–21 Hip joint injection—anterior approach.

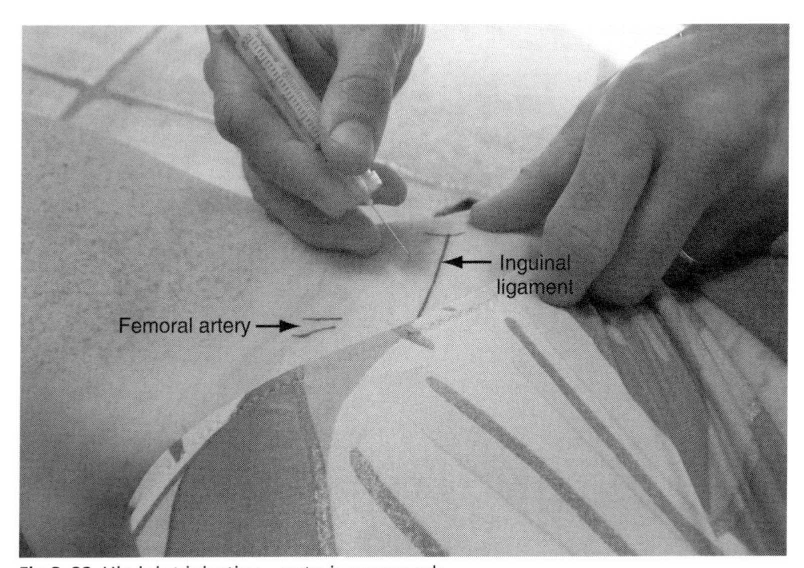

Fig 3–22 Hip joint injection—anterior approach.

their postinjection pain concerns. If there is no relief from the injection, consider other sources of pain (infection, heterotopic ossification, avascular necrosis of the hip, fracture of the hip, Paget's disease, congenital hip dysplasia, referred pain, iliotibial band syndrome, tendinitis). The risk of infection can be minimized with sterile preparation of the area and aseptic technique. Bursitis and/or tendinitis may coexist and may require additional treatment.

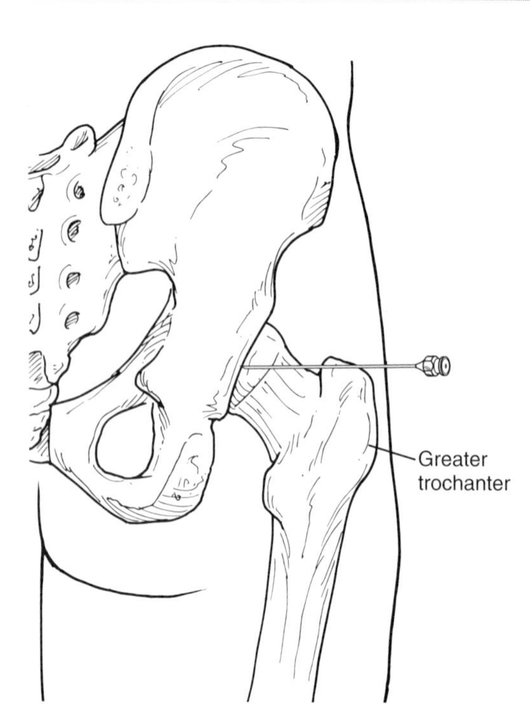

Fig 3–23 Hip joint injection—lateral approach.

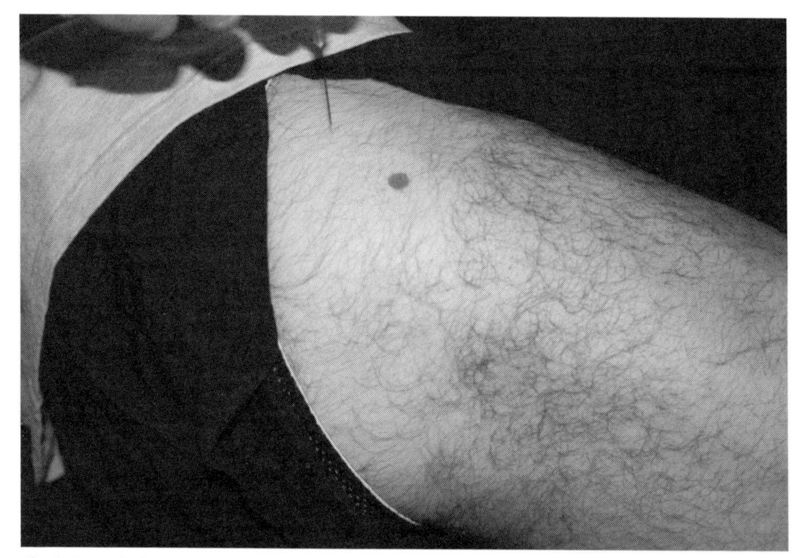

Fig 3–24 Hip joint injection—lateral approach (greater trochanter is marked).

Postinjection Care

Apply a sterile dressing and pressure over the injection site. Have the patient ice the affected area for 20 minutes two to three times daily for the first 24–48 hours. Then begin local heat and gentle stretching exercises several days after the injection. The patient may have improved relief if a 1- to 2-week period of non-weight bearing is initiated on the affected side. Avoid vigorous exercise or running for several days.

When to Perform Follow-Up Injections

Although there are no strict guidelines, a reasonable approach is to reinject in 4–6 weeks if symptoms persist or return. Partial relief of symptoms is an indication for a repeat injection. A total of three injections in a given 12-month period is the accepted standard (hyaluronic acid is given as a series of three to five weekly injections and can be repeated in 6 months). If significant pain relief is not obtained after three injections, consider further imaging studies and possible surgical consultation.

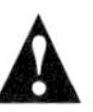

Knee Joint

Name of Procedure

Intraarticular injection of the knee joint is the name of this procedure.

CPT

The Current Procedural Terminology code is 20610 (injection of major joint).

Indications

Intraarticular injections of the knee are usually performed for pain secondary to arthritis (most commonly osteoarthritis or rheumatoid arthritis). Injection is usually offered after a patient has had a course of NSAIDs and/or physical therapy fail and before joint replacement is considered. X-rays (standing AP, lateral, and patellar views) should be taken of the joint before injection.

Symptoms

- Pain localized to the knee.
- Pain worse with activity.
- Decreased functional status in ambulation secondary to pain and decreased range of motion.
- Arthritis in the medial compartment can lead to genu varum (bowleg); arthritis in the lateral compartment can lead to genu valgum (knock-knee).

Physical Examination Findings

- Decreased passive range of motion of the knee joint.
- Crepitus may be noted on range of motion.
- Antalgic gait.
- Quadriceps weakness may be noted (predominantly caused by disuse).
- An effusion may be noted.
- Medial and/or lateral laxity.

Medications to Inject

A corticosteroid and local anesthetic mixture is injected. Some physicians prefer injecting hyaluronic acid.

Amount to Inject

The injectate amount is 5–8 cc.

Size and Gauge of Needle

A 1½–2-inch 21-gauge needle is used. (Needle gauge may vary if aspiration is anticipated.) The length of the needle will depend on how much subcutaneous tissue is in the affected area. People who have more adipose tissue will require the use of a longer needle.

Local Anatomy

The knee joint is composed of the tibiofemoral joint (located between the tibia and the femur) and the patellofemoral joint (located between the patella and the femur).

Patient Position

The patient should be in the supine position.

How and Where to Inject

There are two common approaches for knee injection and aspiration, medial and lateral. These are both retropatellar approaches (between the patella and the femur). Both are performed after Betadine preparation and under aseptic technique. For either approach, the injection site may be first injected with 2–3 mL of 1% lidocaine to provide skin anesthesia.

Lateral Approach

The needle is inserted lateral to the patella at the level of the upper third of the patella anterior to the femur. Medial pressure on the patella can displace the patella laterally and help open the lateral patella space. The needle is directed medially to the retropatellar space between the patella and the lateral femoral condyle. Advance the needle while aspirating. If the needle contacts bone, it should be redirected anteriorly from the femur and posteriorly from the patella. There should be little resistance to injection if the needle is in the joint. If there is resistance, the needle may be in a ligament or tendon, and the position should be changed. Aspirate the joint before injecting to avoid intravascular administration. If aspirate appears infected, do not inject, but send aspirate for analysis. If a large effusion is present, several syringes may be needed to adequately aspirate (Figures 3–25 and 3–26).

Medial Approach

The needle is inserted medial to the patella at the midpoint of the patella. Lateral pressure on the patella will displace it medially and help open the medial space. The needle is directed laterally and slightly cephalad between the patella and the femoral condyle. Advance the needle while aspirating. If the needle contacts bone, it should be redirected anteriorly from the femur and posteriorly from the patella. There should be little resistance to injection if the needle is in the joint. If there is resistance, the needle may be in a ligament or tendon, and the position should be changed. Aspirate the joint before injecting to avoid intravascular administration. If aspirate appears infected, do not inject, but send aspirate for analysis. If a large effusion is present, several syringes may be needed to adequately aspirate (Figures 3–27 and 3–28).

Pitfalls/Complications

Do not inject the joint if acute infection is suspected. It is anticipated that the patient may have an increase in pain for a few days caused by the use of corticosteroids. Informing

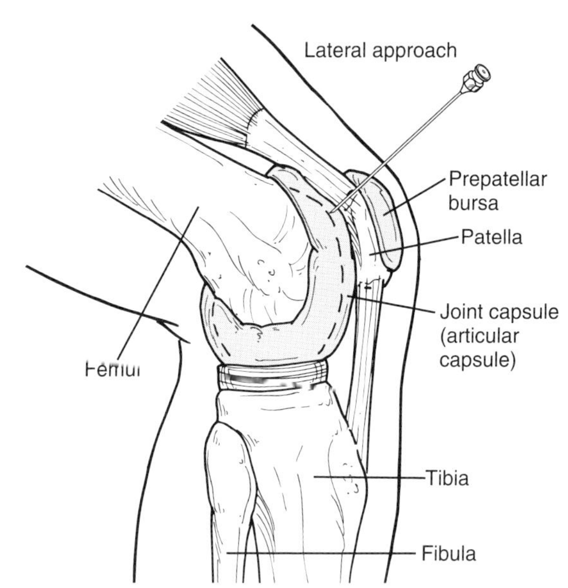

Fig 3–25 Knee joint injection—lateral approach.

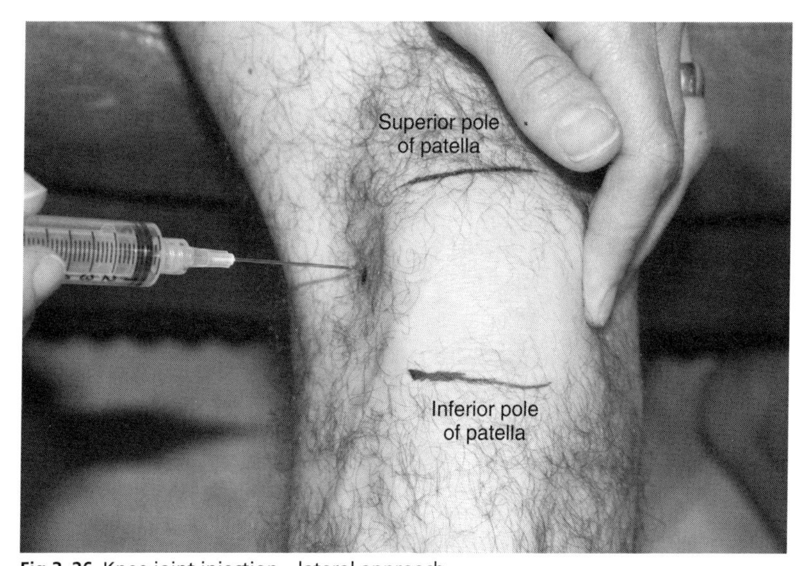

Fig 3–26 Knee joint injection—lateral approach.

patients of this helps to alleviate their postinjection pain concerns. If there is no relief from the injection, consider other sources of pain (fractures, bursitis, tendinitis, infection, internal derangement of the knee, tumor, ankle or hip pathology, osteonecrosis of the tibia or femur). The risk of infection can be minimized with sterile preparation of the area and aseptic technique. Bursitis and/or tendinitis may coexist and may require additional treatment.

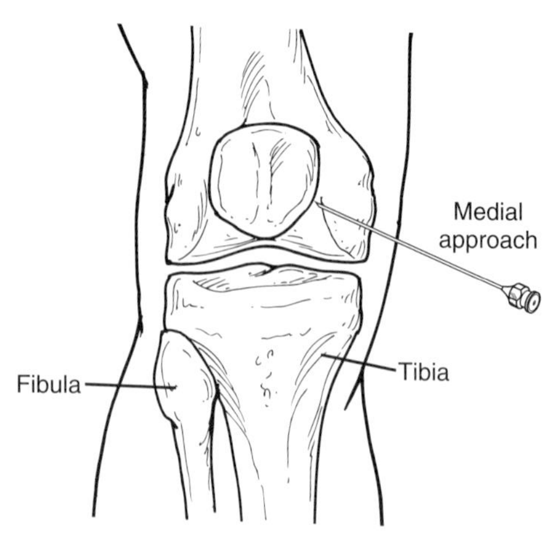

Fig 3–27 Knee joint injection—medial approach.

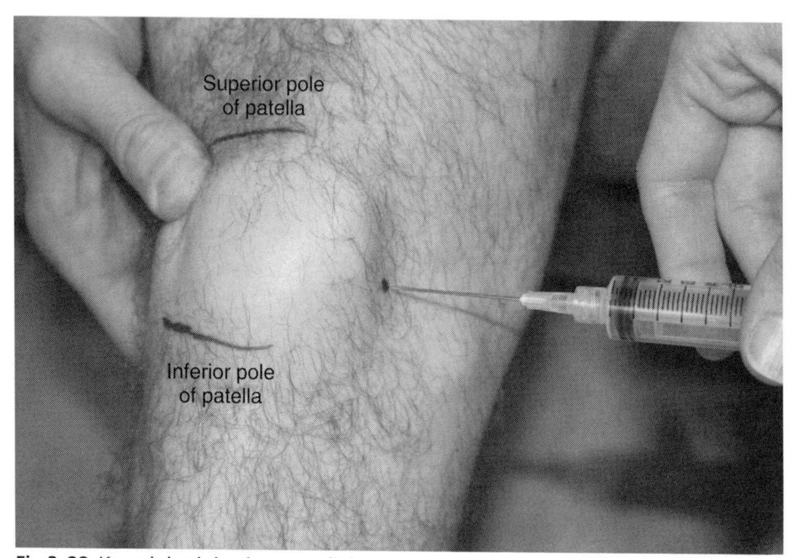

Fig 3–28 Knee joint injection—medial approach.

Postinjection Care

Apply a sterile dressing and pressure over the injection site. Have the patient ice the affected area for 20 minutes two to three times daily for the first 24–48 hours. Then begin local heat and gentle stretching exercises several days after the injection. Straight-leg raising exercises with the knee in extension can be started several days after the injection. Avoid vigorous exercise or running for several days.

When to Perform Follow-Up Injections

Although there are no strict guidelines, a reasonable approach is to reinject in 4–6 weeks if symptoms persist or return. Partial relief of symptoms is an indication for a repeat injection. A total of three injections in a given 12-month period is the accepted standard (hyaluronic acid is given as a series of three to five weekly injections and can be repeated in 6 months). If significant pain relief is not obtained after three injections, consider further imaging studies and possible surgical consultation.

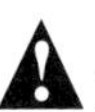

Ankle Joint

Name of Procedure

Intraarticular injection of the ankle joint is the name of this procedure.

CPT

The Current Procedural Terminology code is 20605 (injection of intermediate joint).

Indications

Intraarticular injections of the ankle are usually performed for pain secondary to arthritis (most commonly osteoarthritis, posttraumatic arthritis, or rheumatoid arthritis). Injection is usually offered after a patient has had a course of NSAID, a rigid ankle-foot orthosis, a cane in the opposite hand, and/or physical therapy fail and before joint arthroscopy, arthrodesis, or joint replacement is considered.

Symptoms

- Pain and stiffness localized to the ankle. Pain may radiate to the distal leg.
- Pain worse with activity, especially dorsiflexion.
- Decreased functional status in ambulation secondary to pain and decreased range of motion.

Physical Examination Findings

- Decreased passive range of motion of the joint.
- Deformity of the ankle may be noted.
- Crepitus may be noted on range of motion.
- Antalgic gait.
- Joint swelling and/or tenderness to palpation may be noted.

Medications to Inject

A corticosteroid and local anesthetic mixture is injected. Some physicians prefer injecting hyaluronic acid.

Amount to Inject

The injectate amount is 2–3 mL.

Size and Gauge of Needle

A 1½-inch 23- to 25-gauge needle is used.

Local Anatomy

The ankle articulates the distal tibia, the distal fibula, and the talus. Ligaments (deltoid, anterior talofibular, calcaneofibular, and posterior talofibular) surround the ankle and provide support to the joint.

Patient Position

The patient is supine with the foot in neutral position.

How and Where to Inject

An anteromedial approach should be used (this approach avoids the anterior neurovascular structures). For the anteromedial approach, palpate the tibialis anterior tendon at the level of the distal tibia. A depression should be palpated just medial to the tibialis anterior tendon at the lower margin of the tibia. Mark this area (Figures 3–29 and 3–30). After sterile preparation and with aseptic technique, insert the needle at the marked point. The needle should be directed laterally, perpendicular to the tibia. Inject at a depth of approximately 1–2 cm. If the needle hits the bone, the needle is withdrawn slightly and redirected into the joint space. There should be little resistance to injection if the needle is in the joint. If there is resistance, the needle may be in a ligament or tendon, and the position should be changed. Aspirate the joint before injecting to avoid intravascular administration and to ensure that gross signs of infection are not present.

Pitfalls/Complications

X-rays should be taken of the joint before injection. Do not inject the joint if acute infection is suspected. It is anticipated that the patient may have an increase in pain for a few days caused by the use of corticosteroids. Informing patients of this helps to alleviate their postinjection pain concerns. If there is no relief from the injection, consider other sources of pain (fractures, bursitis, tendinitis, intrinsic instability, ligamentous injury,

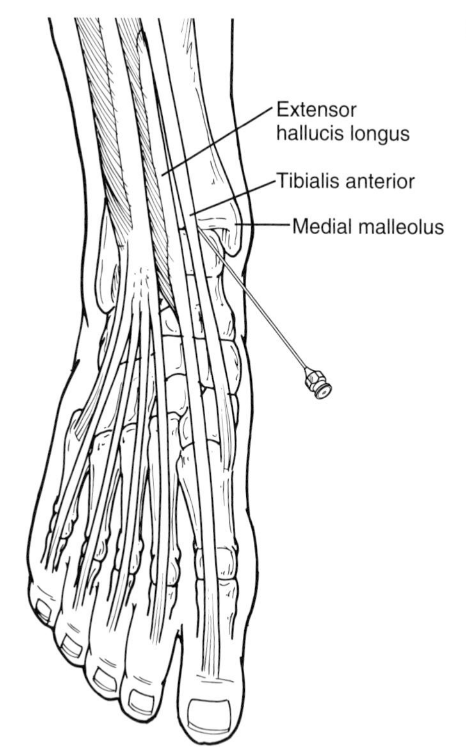

Fig 3–29 Ankle joint injection.

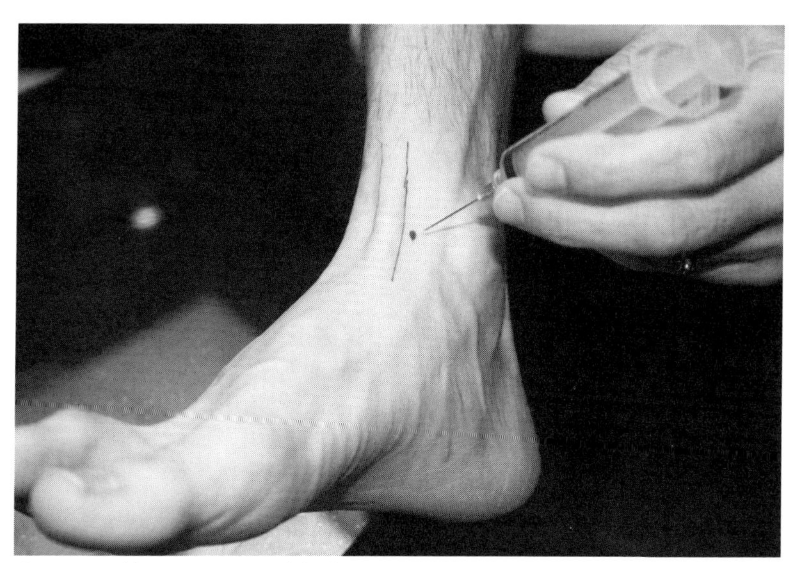

Fig 3–30 Ankle joint injection (tibialis anterior tendon is marked).

infection). The risk of infection can be minimized with Betadine preparation and sterile technique. Bursitis and/or tendinitis may coexist and may require additional treatment.

Postinjection Care

Apply a sterile dressing and pressure over the injection site. Have the patient ice the affected area for 20 minutes two to three times daily for the first 24–48 hours. Then begin local heat and gentle stretching exercises several days after the injection. Avoid vigorous exercise or running for several days.

When to Perform Follow-Up Injections

Although there are no strict guidelines, a reasonable approach is to reinject in 4–6 weeks if symptoms persist or return. Partial relief of symptoms is an indication for a repeat injection. A total of three injections in a given 12-month period is the accepted standard (hyaluronic acid is given as a series of three to five weekly injections and can be repeated in 6 months). If significant pain relief is not obtained after three injections, consider further imaging studies and possible surgical consultation.

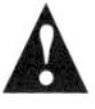

Subtalar Joint

Name of Procedure

Intraarticular injection of the subtalar joint is the name of this procedure.

CPT

The Current Procedural Terminology code is 20605 (injection of intermediate joint).

Indications

Intraarticular injections of the subtalar joint are usually performed for pain secondary to arthritis (most commonly osteoarthritis, but rheumatoid arthritis or posttraumatic arthritis also may respond to injection). Injection is usually offered after a patient has had a course of NSAID and/or physical therapy fail and before surgery is considered.

Symptoms

- Pain within the heel.
- Pain worse with activity such as walking or climbing stairs.
- Decreased functional status in ambulation secondary to pain and decreased range of motion.

Physical Examination Findings

- Decreased passive range of motion of the subtalar joint (decreased passive heel inversion and eversion).
- Crepitus may be noted on range of motion.
- Antalgic gait.
- Increased pain with calcaneal adduction.

Medications to Inject

A corticosteroid and local anesthetic mixture is injected.

Amount to Inject

The injectate amount is 2–3 mL.

Size and Gauge of Needle

A 1½-inch 23- to 25-gauge needle is used.

Local Anatomy

The subtalar joint articulates the talus and the calcaneus. Ligaments (medial and lateral talocalcaneal and interosseous ligaments) surround the ankle and provide support to the joint.

Patient Position

The patient lies supine with the leg slightly abducted and externally rotated so that the medial malleolus is apparent.

How and Where to Inject

A medial or lateral approach can be used.

Medial Approach

The medial malleolus is identified. The sustentaculum tali is a bony protrusion that lies approximately 1 inch below the medial malleolus. The subtalar joint is slightly posterior and cephalad to the sustentaculum tali. Palpate and mark the posterior superior point of the sustentaculum tali. The needle is inserted just posterior and cephalad to this point. Mark this point (Figures 3–31 and 3–32). After sterile preparation and with aseptic technique, the needle is inserted and advanced at a right angle to the ankle. If the needle hits the bone, the needle is withdrawn slightly and redirected into the joint space. There should be little resistance to injection if the needle is in the joint. If there is resistance, the needle may be in a ligament or tendon, and the position should be changed. Aspirate the joint before injecting to ensure that gross signs of infection are not present and to avoid intravascular administration.

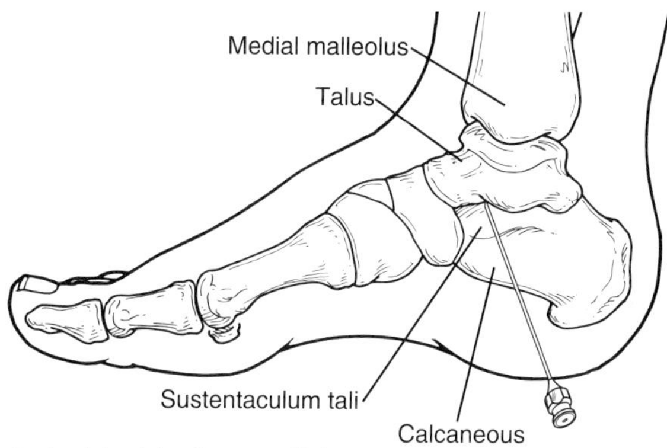

Fig 3–31 Subtalar joint injection—medial approach.

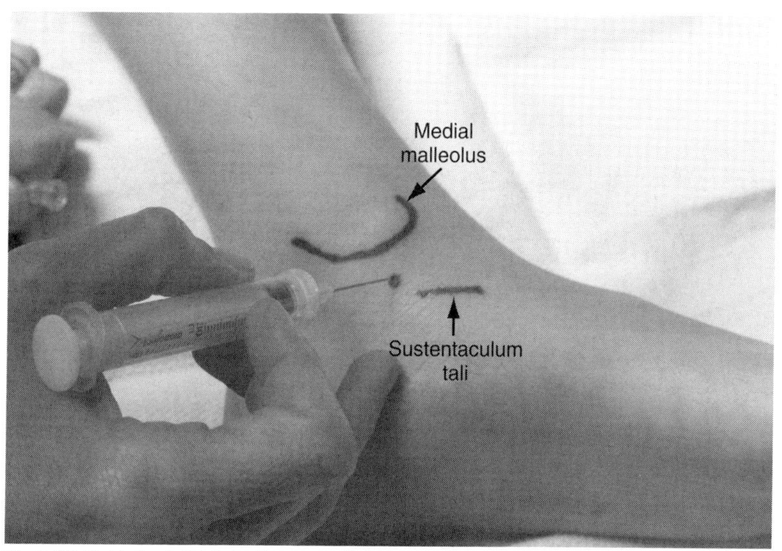

Fig 3–32 Subtalar joint injection—medial approach.

Lateral Approach

The patient lies prone with the feet extending over the end of the table and the foot in neutral position. The needle is directed halfway between the lateral malleolus and the Achilles tendon on a plane parallel to the plantar aspect of the foot. The needle is directed medially and inferiorly toward the medial malleolus. If the needle hits the bone, the needle is withdrawn slightly and redirected into the joint space. There should be little resistance to injection if the needle is in the joint. If there is resistance, the needle may be in a ligament or tendon, and the position should be changed. Aspirate the joint before injecting to ensure that gross signs of infection are not present and to avoid intravascular administration (Figures 3–33 and 3–34).

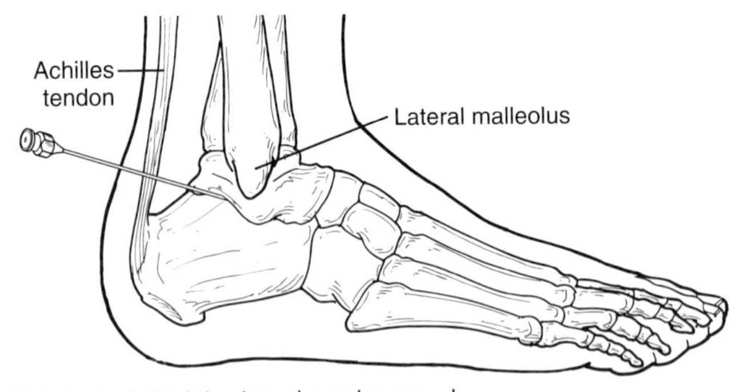

Fig 3–33 Subtalar joint injection—lateral approach.

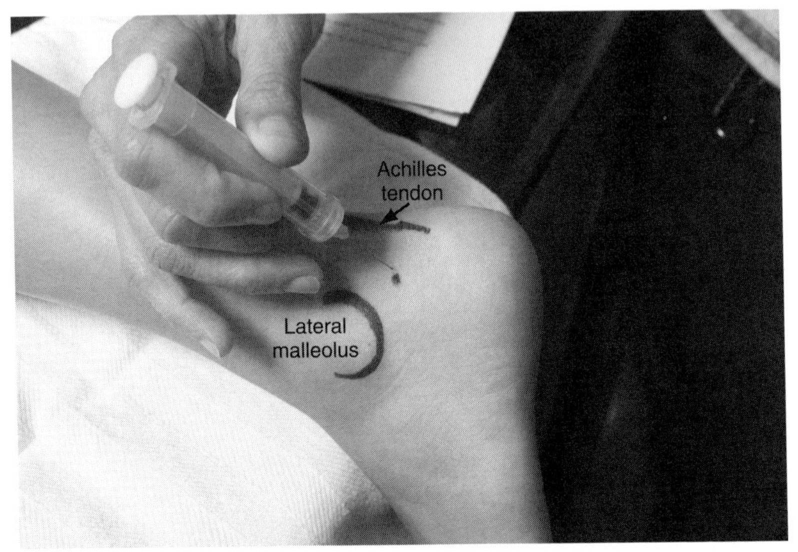

Fig 3–34 Subtalar joint injection—lateral approach.

Pitfalls/Complications

X-rays should be taken of the joint before injection. Do not inject the joint if acute infection is suspected. It is anticipated that the patient may have an increase in pain for a few days caused by the use of corticosteroids. Informing patients of this helps to alleviate their postinjection pain concerns. If there is no relief from the injection, consider other sources of pain (posterior tendon dysfunction, fractures, tendinitis, infection). The risk of infection can be minimized with sterile preparation of the area and aseptic technique. Tendinitis may coexist and may require additional treatment.

Postinjection Care

Apply a sterile dressing and pressure over the injection site. Have the patient ice the affected area for 20 minutes two to three times daily for the first 24–48 hours. Then begin local heat and gentle stretching exercises several days after the injection. Avoid vigorous exercise or running for several days.

When to Perform Follow-Up Injections

Although there are no strict guidelines, a reasonable approach is to reinject in 4–6 weeks if symptoms persist or return. Partial relief of symptoms is an indication for a repeat injection. A total of three injections in a given 12-month period is the accepted standard. If significant pain relief is not obtained after three injections, consider further imaging studies and possible surgical consultation.

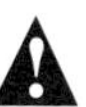

Intertarsal Joint

Name of Procedure

Intraarticular injection of the intertarsal joint is the name of this procedure.

CPT

The Current Procedural Terminology code is 20605 (injection of intermediate joint).

Indications

Intraarticular injections of the intertarsal joint are usually performed for pain secondary to arthritis (most commonly osteoarthritis, but rheumatoid arthritis or posttraumatic arthritis may also respond to injection). Injection is usually offered after a patient has had a course of NSAID and/or physical therapy fail.

Symptoms

- Pain localized to the dorsum of the foot.
- Pain worse with inversion and adduction of the midtarsal joints.

Physical Examination Findings

- Decreased passive range of motion of the joint, especially inversion and adduction.
- Crepitus may be noted on range of motion.
- Decreased functional ability in walking and climbing stairs may be noted.

Medications to Inject

A corticosteroid and local anesthetic mixture (do not use anesthetic with epinephrine) is injected.

Amount to Inject

The injectate amount is 2–3 mL.

Size and Gauge of Needle

A ⅝-inch 25-gauge needle is used.

Local Anatomy

The intertarsal bones articulate with each other and the metatarsals.

Patient Position

The patient is in the supine position.

How and Where to Inject

The most tender area of the intertarsal joint is identified (generally at the midtarsal level between the navicular and cuneiform bones, hence midtarsal joint). Palpate and mark the articulation of greatest tenderness. The needle is inserted at a right angle to the dorsal aspect of the foot at this point. Some physicians prefer to do the injection under fluoroscopic guidance for precise localization. If the needle contacts the bone, the needle is withdrawn slightly and redirected into the joint space. There should be little resistance to injection if the needle is in the joint. If there is resistance, the needle may be in a ligament or tendon, and the position should be changed. Aspirate the joint before injecting and avoid intravascular administration (Figures 3–35 and 3–36).

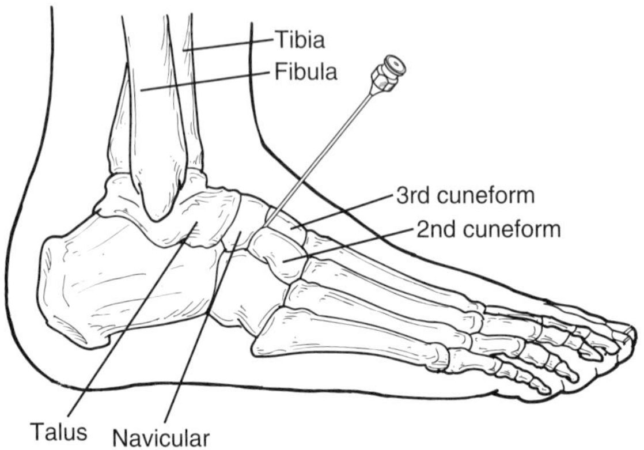

Fig 3–35 Intertarsal joint injection.

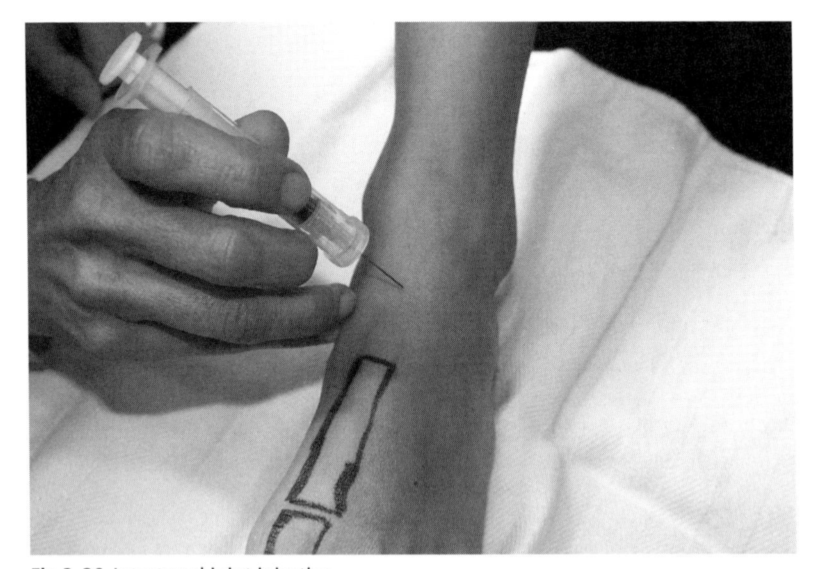

Fig 3–36 Intertarsal joint injection.

Pitfalls/Complications

X-rays should be taken of the joint before injection. Do not inject the joint if acute infection is suspected. It is anticipated that the patient may have an increase in pain for a few days caused by the use of corticosteroids. Informing patients of this helps to alleviate their postinjection pain concerns. If there is no relief from the injection, consider other sources of pain (fractures, avascular necrosis, tendinitis, infection). The risk of infection can be minimized with sterile preparation of the area and aseptic technique. Tendinitis may coexist and may require additional treatment.

Postinjection Care

Apply a sterile dressing and pressure over the injection site. Have the patient ice the affected area for 20 minutes two to thee times daily for the first 24–48 hours. Then begin local heat and gentle stretching exercises several days after the injection. Avoid vigorous exercise or running for several days.

When to Perform Follow-Up Injections

Although there are no strict guidelines, a reasonable approach is to reinject in 4–6 weeks if symptoms persist or return. If no relief is obtained under initial injection, consider performing repeat injections under fluoroscopic guidance. Partial relief of symptoms is an indication for a repeat injection. A total of three injections in a given 12-month period is the accepted standard. If significant pain relief is not obtained after three injections, consider further imaging studies and possible surgical consultation.

Metatarsophalangeal Joint

Name of Procedure

Intraarticular injection of the metatarsophalangeal joint is the name of this procedure.

CPT

The Current Procedural Terminology code is 20600 (injection of small joint).

Indications

Intraarticular injections of the metatarsophalangeal joint are usually performed for pain secondary to arthritis (most commonly osteoarthritis or rheumatoid arthritis) or gout. The first metatarsophalangeal joint is most commonly affected. Injection is usually offered after a patient has had a course of NSAID and orthotics fail.

Symptoms

- Pain and stiffness localized to the metatarsophalangeal joint.
- In gout, patient may complain of severe pain in the metatarsophalangeal joint, which may be swollen and painful.
- Pain worse with activity, especially the toe-off phase of gait.
- Decreased functional status in ambulation secondary to pain and decreased range of motion.
- Bony changes may be present in advanced gout.

Physical Examination Findings

- Decreased passive range of motion of the joint, especially loss of extension of the joint.
- Crepitus may be noted on range of motion.

- Pain on dorsiflexion of the joint.
- Antalgic gait.
- In patients with gout, the joint may be swollen and tender.

Medications to Inject

A corticosteroid and local anesthetic mixture is injected.

Amount to Inject

The injectate amount is 1½–2 mL.

Size and Gauge of Needle

A ⅝-inch 25- or 27-gauge needle is used.

Local Anatomy

The metatarsophalangeal joint lies between the metatarsals and the phalanges in each of the toes. Ligaments surround the joints and help to strengthen them.

Patient Position

The patient is in the supine position with the foot placed on the table.

How and Where to Inject

A dorsal approach is used. Palpate the margins of the metatarsophalangeal joint with the toe in plantar flexion. The needle is inserted into the joint. If the needle hits the bone, the needle is withdrawn slightly and redirected into the joint space. There should be little resistance to injection if the needle is in the joint. If there is resistance, the needle may be in a ligament or tendon, and the position should be changed. Aspiration should be performed if gout is suspected, and the joint aspirate should be sent for analysis. Aspirate before injecting to avoid intravascular administration and to ensure no gross signs of infection (Figures 3–37 and 3–38).

Pitfalls/Complications

X-rays should be taken of the joint before injection. Do not inject the joint if acute infection is suspected. Acute gout may present with a hot red swollen joint and may mimic

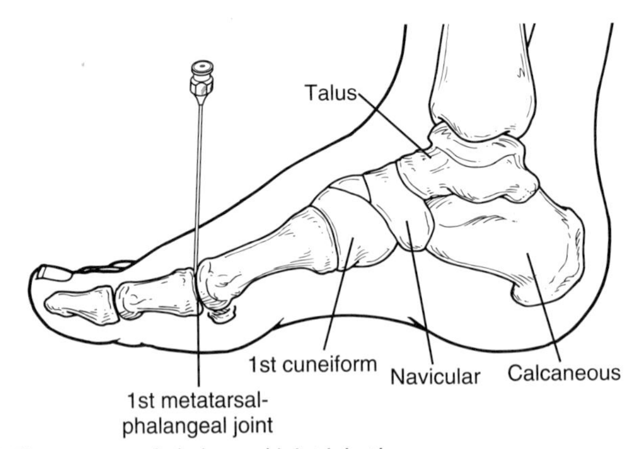

Fig 3–37 First metatarsal phalangeal joint injection.

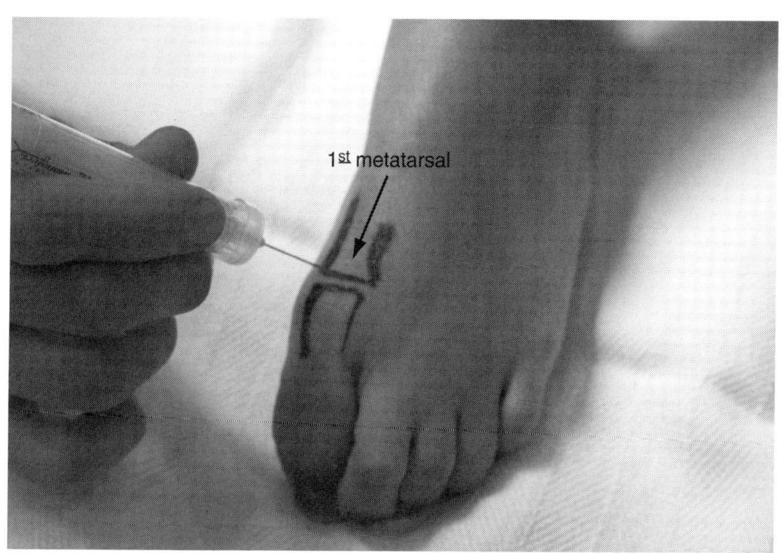

Fig 3–38 First metatarsal phalangeal joint injection.

infection. It is anticipated that the patient may have an increase in pain for a few days caused by the use of corticosteroids. Informing patients of this helps to alleviate their postinjection pain concerns. If there is no relief from the injection, consider other sources of pain (fractures, tendinitis, infection). The risk of infection can be minimized with sterile preparation of the area and aseptic technique. Tendinitis may coexist and may require additional treatment.

Postinjection Care

Apply a sterile dressing and pressure over the injection site. Have the patient ice the affected area for 20 minutes two to three times daily for the first 24–48 hours. Then begin local heat and gentle stretching exercises several days after the injection. Avoid vigorous exercise or running for several days. Encourage use of a shoe with a solid sole and wide toebox.

When to Perform Follow-Up Injections

Although there are no strict guidelines, a reasonable approach is to reinject in 4–6 weeks if symptoms persist or return. Partial relief of symptoms is an indication for a repeat injection. A total of three injections in a given 12-month period is the accepted standard. If significant pain relief is not obtained after three injections, consider further imaging studies and possible surgical consultation.

4

Tendons

The injection procedures here are based on a review of the various techniques described in the medical literature as well as the authors' experiences. The techniques chosen are felt to be the most appropriate in most cases. As clinical circumstances may differ, other approaches may be more appropriate for individual cases. The reader is encouraged to familiarize himself/herself with the additional sources in the bibliography at the end of this chapter for additional approaches.

All procedures should be performed using appropriate preparation and aseptic technique. Local anesthesia (either injected or vapo-coolant spray) may be helpful in most procedures. As always, the clinician should weigh the risks and benefits of any interventional procedure.

Trigger Finger (Stenosing Flexor Tenosynovitis)

Name of Procedure

Injection of trigger finger (stenosing flexor tenosynovitis) is the name of this procedure.

CPT

The Current Procedural Terminology code is 20550 (injection of tendon sheath).

Indications

This can be a firstline treatment for trigger finger, or it can be a treatment offered after a patient has had a course of NSAID, buddy taping to the next finger, and/or physical/occupational therapy.

Symptoms

- Locking or catching (triggering) of the finger as it is flexed and extended.
- Pain in the proximal interphalangeal joint, the metacarpophalangeal joint, or in the distal palm.
- Finger may become locked in one position.
- May have a tender nodule that is palpable.
- May complain of swelling and/or stiffness in the fingers.
- Pain worse with activities that require gripping.
- More common in patients with diabetes or rheumatoid arthritis.
- May require external force to straighten the finger.

Physical Examination Findings

- Triggering of the finger.
- May have a tender nodule that is palpable.

- May have decreased range of motion of the finger caused by pain or contractures.
- With the metacarpal phalangeal joint flexed, the joint may be flexed passively without pain.

Medications to Inject

A corticosteroid and local anesthetic mixture (do not use anesthetic with epinephrine) is injected.

Amount to Inject

The injectate amount is 1–2 mL.

Size and Gauge of Needle

A $\frac{5}{8}$–1-inch 25- to 27-gauge needle is used.

Local Anatomy

The tendons of the finger flexors are inflamed and swollen, usually secondary to compression by the heads of the metacarpal bones. This usually occurs at the level of the metacarpal heads. The inflammation and swelling can become chronic and result in a thickening of the tendon sheath. A nodule may develop on the tendon, which may be palpated when the patient flexes and extends the finger. The triggering phenomenon is caused when the nodule catches in the tendon sheath as the nodule passes under the A1 pulley at the metacarpal head.

Patient Position

The arm should be adducted at the side and the hand held palm up (usually with a towel under the dorsum of the hand)

How and Where to Inject

After Betadine prep and with aseptic technique, insert the needle at a 45-degree angle parallel to the affected tendon (usually proximal to the distal volar crease in the midline) (Figures 4–1 and 4–2). Direct the needle toward the swollen nodule of the tendon. If the

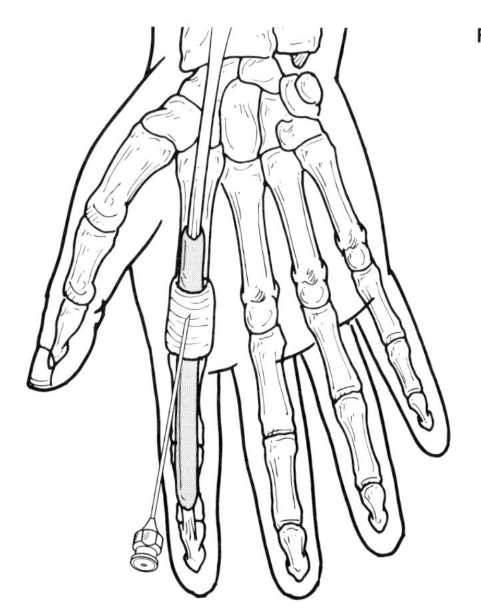

Fig 4–1 Trigger finger injection.

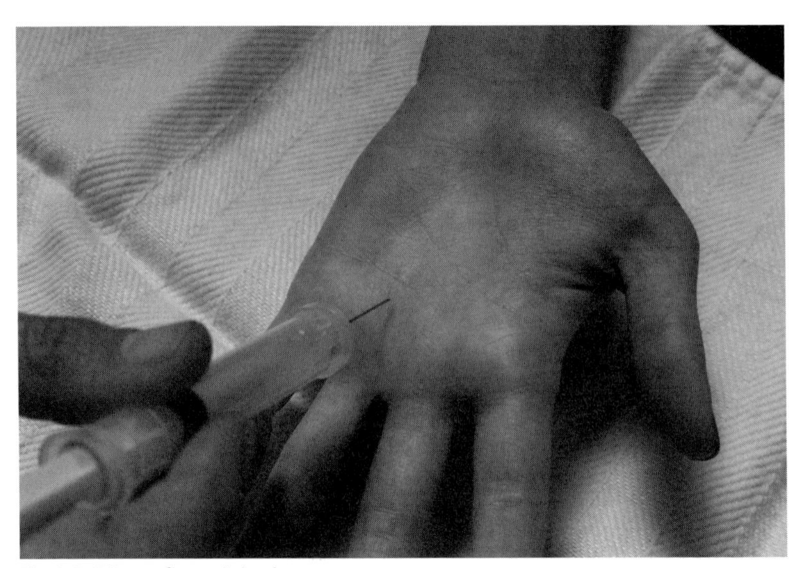

Fig 4–2 Trigger finger injection.

needle hits the bone, the needle is withdrawn slightly. If the needle is in the tendon, it will move with finger movement. The needle should be withdrawn slightly so that it is in the tendon sheath and not the tendon. If there is resistance, the needle may be in a ligament or tendon, and the position should be changed. Aspirate before injecting to ensure that infection is not present and to avoid intravascular administration.

Pitfalls/Complications

It is anticipated that the patient may have an increase in pain for a few days caused by the use of corticosteroids. Informing patients of this helps to alleviate their postinjection pain concerns. If there is no relief from the injection, consider other sources of pain (joint instability, fracture, anomalous muscle belly in the palm, ganglion or tumor of the tendon sheath, rheumatoid arthritis). The risk of infection can be minimized with sterile preparation of the area and aseptic technique. Injections directly into the tendon may increase the likelihood of tendon rupture and should be avoided. Because patients with rheumatoid arthritis are more prone to tendon rupture, they may be referred for surgical release after only one injection. Occasionally, subcutaneous atrophy and loss of pigmentation can occur.

Postinjection Care

Apply a sterile dressing and pressure over the injection site. Have the patient ice the affected area for 20 minutes two to three times daily for the first 24–48 hours. Then begin local heat and gentle stretching exercises several days after the injection. Avoid vigorous exercise or use of the hand for several days. A hand splint (with the MCP joint in 10–15 degrees) to protect the fingers may help to relieve the symptoms.

When to Perform Follow-Up Injections

Although there are no strict guidelines, a reasonable approach is to reinject in 4–6 weeks if symptoms persist or return. Partial relief of symptoms is an indication for a repeat injection. A total of three injections in a given 12-month period is the accepted standard.

If significant pain relief is not obtained after three injections, consider further imaging studies and possible surgical consultation.

De Quervain's (Tenosynovitis of the Wrist)

Name of Procedure

De Quervain's injection for de Quervain's tenosynovitis (stenosing tenosynovitis of the first dorsal wrist compartment) is the name for this procedure.

CPT

The Current Procedural Terminology code is 20550 (injection of tendon sheath).

Indications

This can be a firstline treatment for de Quervain's tenosynovitis, or it can be a treatment offered after a patient has had a course of immobilization of the thumb in a thumb spica splint and/or NSAID.

Symptoms

- Pain and swelling over the radial styloid.
- Aggravation of symptoms with thumb movement and/or ulnar deviation of the wrist.
- Patient may complain of triggering or sticking of the tendons as the thumb is moved.
- Pain with lifting with the forearms in a neutral position between pronation and supination (frequently seen in mothers of pre-toddlers, who are repeatedly lifting their children out of cribs).

Physical Examination Findings

- Swelling over the distal radius in the synovial compartment.
- Pain on resisted thumb extension.
- Positive Finkelstein test (pain reproduced with ulnar dev iation of the wrist while the thumb is flexed into the palm).
- Crepitus may be noted as the patient flexes and extends the thumb.
- Triggering or sticking of the tendons as the patient moves the thumb.

Medications to Inject

A corticosteroid and local anesthetic mixture is injected.

Amount to Inject

The injectate amount is 1–3 mL.

Size and Gauge of Needle

A $\frac{7}{8}$-inch 25- to 27-gauge needle is used.

Local Anatomy

The tendons of the abductor pollicis longus and extensor pollicis brevis are located in the first dorsal wrist compartment just distal to the radial styloid. Two discreet tendons can be palpated traveling together. The superficial branch of the radial nerve and the radial artery are located medially (toward the palmar side).

Patient Position

Have the patient rest his/her wrist comfortably on the table with the radial side facing up and the ulnar surface of the wrist slightly elevated on a towel to relax the tendons.

How and Where to Inject

If possible, inject between the tendons of the abductor pollicis longus and extensor pollicis brevis (just distal to the radial styloid) (Figures 4–3 and 4–4). Alternately, inject in the sheath around both of these tendons. Once the needle is in, ask the patient to move his/her thumb. If the needle moves with the thumb, you are in the tendon. Pull the needle back approximately 1mm so that you are in the tendon sheath and not the tendon. If there is resistance, the needle may be in a ligament or tendon, and the position should be changed. A small swelling along the length of the tendon indicates that the injection is in the tendon sheath. Aspirate before injecting to avoid intravascular administration.

Pitfalls/Complications

It is anticipated that the patient may have an increase in pain for a few days caused by the use of corticosteroids. Informing patients of this helps to alleviate their postinjection pain concerns. If there is no relief from the injection, consider other sources of pain (arthritis of the thumb, fracture of the scaphoid, trigger thumb, gout, superficial radial neuropathy, cervical radiculopathy). Injury to the radial sensory nerve is possible during the injection. If the patient complains of tingling in a radial distribution during the injection, reposition the needle. The superficial branch of the radial nerve and the radial artery can be traumatized if the needle is placed too medially. Occasionally, subcutaneous atrophy and loss of pigmentation can occur. The risk of infection can be minimized with sterile preparation of the area and aseptic technique. Injections directly into the tendon may increase the likelihood of tendon rupture and should be avoided.

Postinjection Care

Apply a sterile dressing and pressure over the injection site. Have the patient ice the affected area for 20 minutes two to three times daily for the first 24–48 hours. A thumb spica splint should be used at night for the first week. Avoid strenuous use of the hand and wrist for several days.

When to Perform Follow-Up Injections

Although there are no strict guidelines, a reasonable approach is to reinject in 4–6 weeks if symptoms persist or return. Partial relief of symptoms is an indication for a repeat injection. A total of three injections in a given 12-month period is the accepted standard. If significant pain relief is not obtained after three injections, consider further imaging studies and possible surgical consultation.

Bicipital Tendinitis

Name of Procedure

This procedure is called injection of biceps tendon for bicipital tendinitis. Although this is commonly referred to as a tendinitis, a more accurate description may be tendinosis because signs of inflammation may be absent.

CPT

The Current Procedural Terminology code is 20550 (injection of tendon sheath).

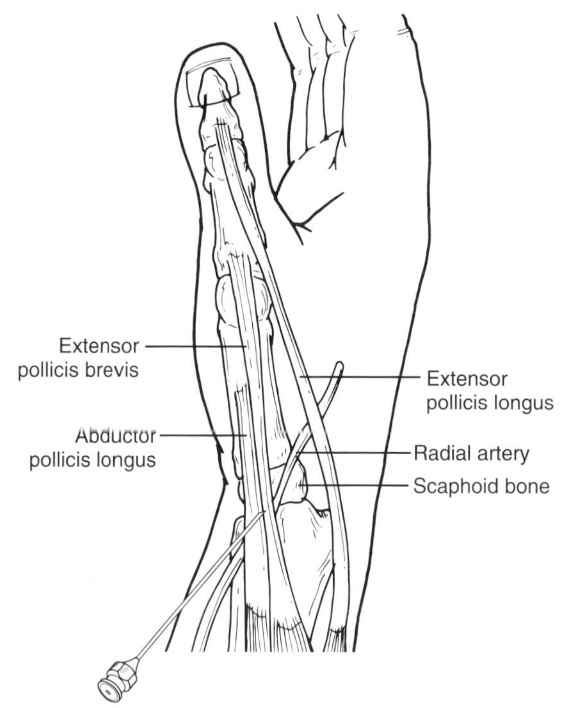

Fig 4–3 de Quervain's injection.

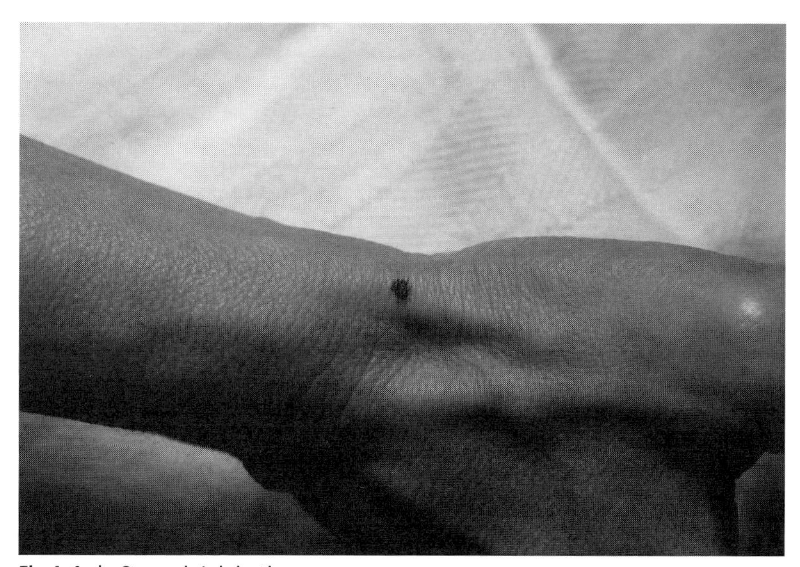

Fig 4–4 de Quervain's injection.

Indications

This injection is usually used for bicipital tendinitis after a patient has failed a course of NSAID and/or physical therapy.

Symptoms

- Pain in the anterior shoulder over the bicipital groove, worse with activity.
- Patient may feel a "catching" sensation with overhead activities, especially with elbow flexion.
- Decreased functional ability secondary to decreased range of motion of the shoulder.

Physical Examination Findings

- Positive Yergason sign (pain in the bicipital groove with resisted supination of the forearm with the elbow flexed to 90 degrees).
- Positive Speed's test (pain in the bicipital groove with resisted forward shoulder flexion with the elbow in extension and the forearm in supination).
- Palpable tenderness over the bicipital groove.
- After prolonged periods, muscle wasting or a frozen shoulder may be noted.

Medications to Inject

A corticosteroid and local anesthetic mixture is injected.

Amount to Inject

The injectate amount is 1–3 mL.

Size and Gauge of Needle

A 1–1½-inch 25- to 27-gauge needle is used.

Local Anatomy

The long head of the biceps muscle originates in the supraglenoid tubercle of the scapula. The short head of the biceps originates from the tip of the coracoid process of the scapula. The biceps tendons (either the long head, the short head, or both) can become impinged at the coracoacromial arch. In addition, this is a "watershed" area, where there is limited vascular supply to the tendons. Tendinitis of the biceps may coexist with shoulder bursitis and impingement. The tendon of the long head of the biceps may rupture, resulting in balling of the muscle distally.

Patient Position

The affected arm is externally rotated 45 degrees. The coracoid process is identified anteriorly.

How and Where to Inject

The biceps tendon is palpated in the anterior shoulder approximately 1–1¼ inches below the anterolateral aspect of the acromion, over the bicipital groove (Figures 4–5 and 4–6). The bevel of the needle should be parallel to the fibers of the tendon. Once the needle is in, ask the patient to flex the elbow. If the needle moves with the elbow, you are in the tendon. Retract the needle 1 mm so that you are in the tendon sheath and not the tendon. If there is resistance, the needle may be in a ligament or tendon, and the position should be changed. Aspirate before injecting to ensure that infection is not present and to avoid intravascular administration.

Pitfalls/Complications

It is anticipated that the patient may have an increase in pain for a few days caused by the use of corticosteroids. Informing patients of this helps to alleviate their postinjection

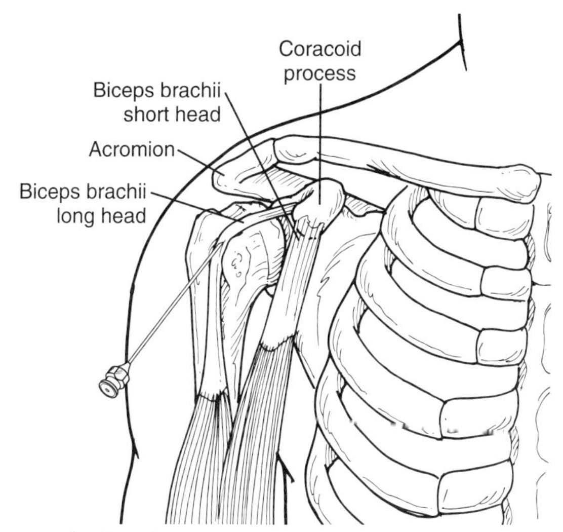

Fig 4–5 Biceps tendon injection.

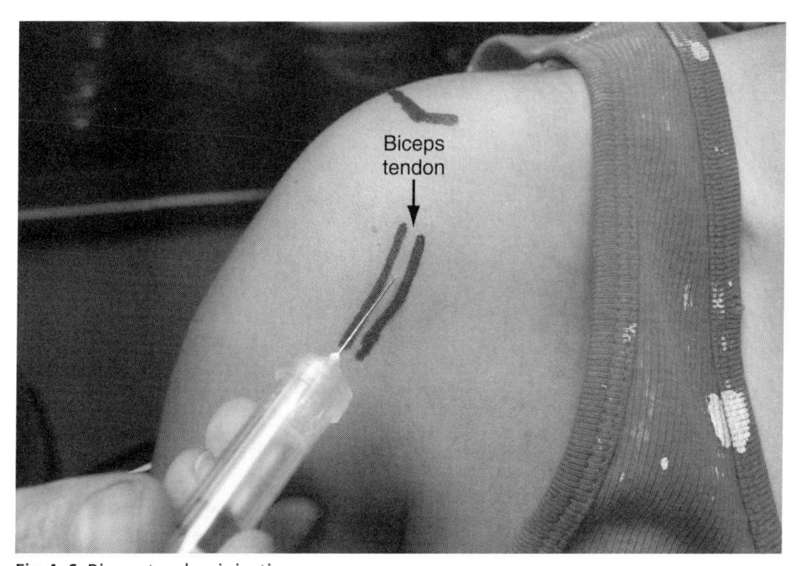

Fig 4–6 Biceps tendon injection.

pain concerns. If there is no relief from the injection, consider other sources of pain (impingement syndrome, biceps tendon rupture, adhesive capsulitis, cervical spondylosis, cervical radiculopathy, shoulder arthritis, thoracic outlet syndrome, brachial plexopathy). Occasionally, subcutaneous atrophy and loss of pigmentation can occur. The risk of infection can be minimized with sterile preparation of the area and aseptic technique. Injections directly into the tendon may increase the likelihood of tendon rupture and should be avoided.

Postinjection Care

Apply a sterile dressing and pressure over the injection site. Have the patient ice the affected area for 20 minutes two to three times daily for the first 24–48 hours. Then begin local heat and gentle stretching exercises several days after the injection. Avoid vigorous exercise or overhead use of the arm for several days. Isometric elbow flexion exercises may be begun after pain has subsided.

When to Perform Follow-Up Injections

Although there are no strict guidelines, a reasonable approach is to reinject in 4–6 weeks if symptoms persist or return. Partial relief of symptoms is an indication for a repeat injection. A total of three injections in a given 12-month period is the accepted standard. If significant pain relief is not obtained after three injections, consider further imaging studies and possible surgical consultation.

Lateral Epicondylitis

Name of Procedure

This procedure is called injection of the lateral epicondyle. Although this is commonly referred to as a tendinitis, a more accurate description may be tendinosis, because signs of inflammation are usually absent (also referred to as tennis elbow).

CPT

The Current Procedural Terminology code is 20550 (injection of tendon sheath).

Indications

Injection treatment is usually offered after a patient has had a course of NSAID, a tennis elbow strap (worn just below the elbow), and/or physical therapy.

Symptoms

- Frequently seen in repetitive overuse activities of the arms.
- Pain on the lateral aspect of the elbow and the back of the upper forearm.
- Increased pain with lifting, especially when lifting with the palm facing down.
- Pain with wrist or hand movements (griping or carrying).

Physical Examination Findings

- Pain on palpation of the wrist extensor muscles (just distal to the lateral epicondyle).
- Pain on resisted wrist extension (especially if the elbow is extended, the forearm pronated, the wrist radially deviated, and the hand in a fist).
- Pain over the lateral epicondyle with resisted extension of the proximal interphalangeal joint of the long finger.
- Pain may radiate proximally or distally.
- May be swelling over the lateral epicondyle.
- May note diminished grip strength.

Medications to Inject

A corticosteroid and local anesthetic mixture is injected.

Amount to Inject

The injectate amount is 2–6 mL.

Size and Gauge of Needle

A 1-inch 25-gauge needle is used.

Local Anatomy

Microtears can occur at the origin of the extensor carpi radialis brevis (most likely), the extensor carpi radialis longus, and/or the extensor digitorum communis muscles over the anterior facet of the lateral epicondyle.

Patient Position

The arm should be against the chest (fully adducted), the elbow should be flexed to 90 degrees, and the forearm should be pronated.

How and Where to Inject

Inject near the extensor carpi radialis brevis tendon, palpated 1–5 cm distal to the lateral epicondyle (Figures 4–7 and 4–8). The medication should be placed at the interface of the subcutaneous fat and the tendon. This should be the area of maximum tenderness. If resistance is encountered, the needle may be in the tendon. Withdraw the needle until no significant resistance is encountered. The goal is to inject in the region of the tendon but not in the tendon itself. Because of the large area of the extensor tendon origin, a "peppering" technique (injecting small amounts at a time in a larger area), rather than a large bolus, may be beneficial. Aspirate before injecting to ensure that infection is not present and to avoid intravascular administration.

Pitfalls/Complications

It is anticipated that the patient may have an increase in pain for a few days caused by the use of corticosteroids. Informing patients of this helps to alleviate their postinjection pain concerns. If there is no relief from the injection, consider other sources of

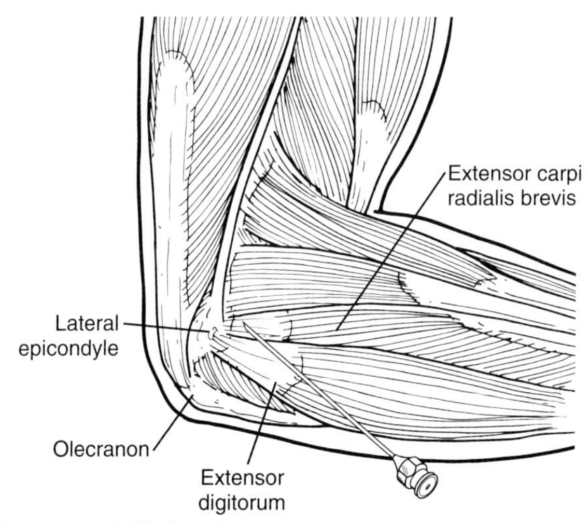

Fig 4–7 Lateral epicondylitis injection.

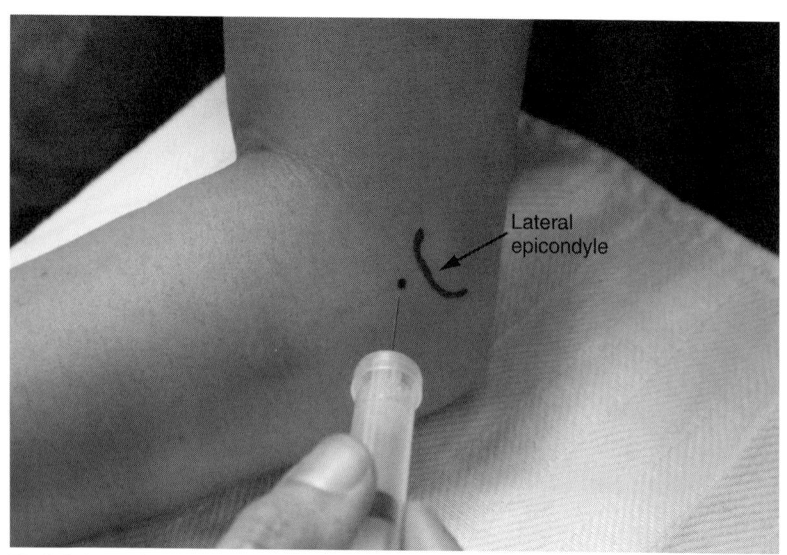

Fig 4–8 Lateral epicondylitis injection.

pain (radial tunnel syndrome, cervical radiculopathy, arthritis, fracture, radial nerve irritation in the forearm, triceps tendinitis, bursitis, elbow synovitis). The risk of infection can be minimized with sterile preparation of the area and aseptic technique. Occasionally, subcutaneous atrophy and loss of pigmentation can occur. Injections directly into the tendon may increase the likelihood of tendon rupture and should be avoided.

Postinjection Care

Apply a sterile dressing and pressure over the injection site. Have the patient ice the affected area for 20 minutes two to three times daily for the first 24–48 hours. A wrist splint can be used for several days. Then begin local heat and gentle stretching exercises several days after the injection. Avoid vigorous exercise or heavy lifting for several days. Isometric gripping exercises and wrist extension exercises may be begun after symptoms have improved. If the cause of epicondylitis was a racquet sport, check the weight, handle size, and stringing of the racquet and evaluate the patient's stroke so that the disorder does not recur. Check for recent restringing, change of racquet, or increased frequency of play as causative factors of an overuse injury.

When to Perform Follow-Up Injections

Although there are no strict guidelines, a reasonable approach is to reinject in 4–6 weeks if symptoms persist or return. Partial relief of symptoms is an indication for a repeat injection. A total of three injections in a given 12-month period is the accepted standard. Botox into the extensor muscles has been reported to be beneficial if cortico-steroid/local anesthetic injections do not provide relief. If significant pain relief is not obtained after three injections, consider further imaging studies and possible surgical consultation.

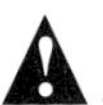

Medial Epicondylitis

Name of Procedure

This procedure is called injection of the medial epicondyle. Although this is commonly referred to as a tendinitis, a more accurate description may be tendinosis because signs of inflammation are usually absent (also referred to as golfer's elbow).

CPT

The Current Procedural Terminology code is 20550 (injection of tendon sheath).

Indications

Injection treatment is usually offered after a patient has had a course of NSAID, an elbow strap (worn just below the elbow), and/or physical therapy.

Symptoms

- Frequently seen in repetitive overuse activities of the arms.
- Pain on the medial aspect of the elbow and the upper forearm.
- Increased pain with lifting.
- Pain with wrist or hand movements.

Physical Examination Findings

- Pain on palpation of the wrist flexor muscles (just distal to the medial epicondyle).
- Pain over the medial epicondyle with resisted wrist flexion.
- Pain may radiate proximally or distally.
- May be swelling over the medial epicondyle.
- May note diminished grip strength.

Medications to Inject

A corticosteroid and local anesthetic mixture is injected.

Amount to Inject

The injectate amount is 2–6 mL.

Size and Gauge of Needle

A 1-inch 25-gauge needle is used.

Local Anatomy

Microtears can occur at the origin of the flexor carpi radialis and flexor carpi ulnaris muscles near the medial epicondyle.

Patient Position

The arm should be against the chest (fully adducted), the elbow should be flexed to 90 degrees, and the forearm should be supinated.

How and Where to Inject

Inject near the flexor forearm muscles, palpated 1–5 cm distal to the medial epicondyle (Figures 4–9 and 4–10). The medication should be placed at the interface of the subcutaneous fat and the tendon. This should be the area of maximum tenderness. If resistance

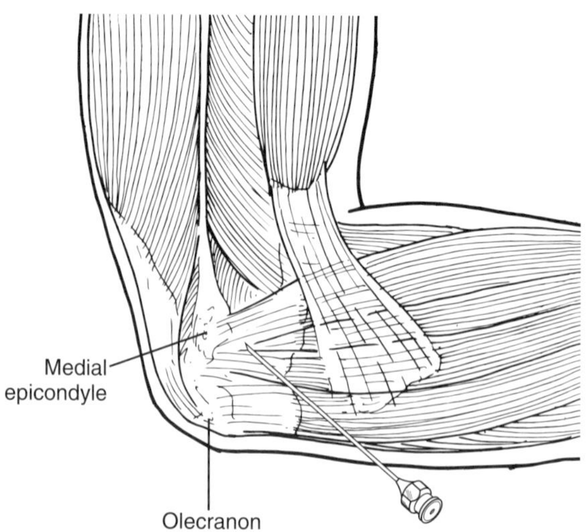

Fig 4–9 Medial epicondylitis injection.

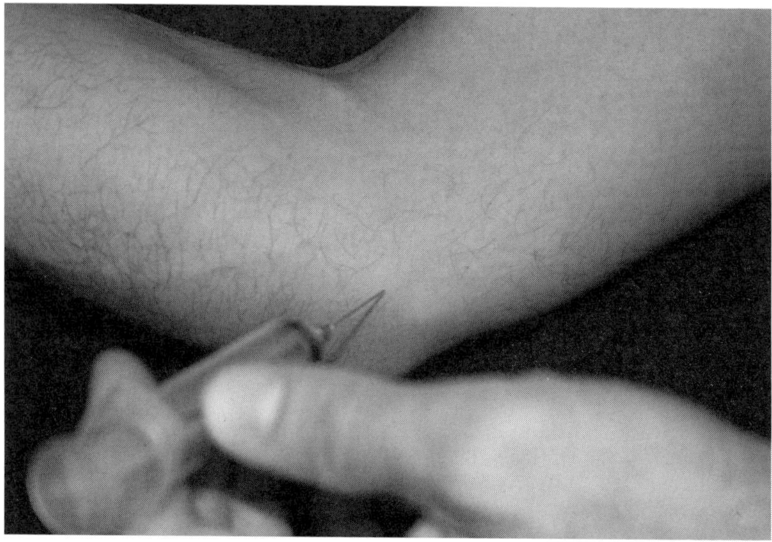

Fig 4–10 Medial epicondylitis injection.

is encountered, the needle may be in the tendon. Withdraw the needle until no significant resistance is encountered. The goal is to inject into the region of the tendon but not in the tendon itself; a "peppering" technique (injecting small amounts at a time in a larger area), rather than a large bolus, may be beneficial. Aspirate before injecting to ensure that infection is not present and to avoid intravascular administration.

Pitfalls/Complications

It is anticipated that the patient may have an increase in pain for a few days caused by the use of corticosteroids. Informing patients of this helps to alleviate their postinjection pain concerns. If there is no relief from the injection, consider other sources of pain (ulnar neuropathy, cervical radiculopathy, arthritis, fracture, triceps tendinitis, common flexor tendon avulsion, bursitis, elbow synovitis). The risk of infection can be minimized with sterile preparation of the area and aseptic technique. Occasionally, subcutaneous atrophy and loss of pigmentation can occur. Because the ulnar nerve is close to this area, the patient should be warned of possible dysesthesias or paresthesia. If these are noted during needle insertion, the needle should be immediately withdrawn from the nerve. Spread of the local anesthetic may cause a temporary ulnar nerve block, and the patient should also be aware of this possibility. Injections directly into the tendon may increase the likelihood of tendon rupture and should be avoided.

Postinjection Care

Apply a sterile dressing and pressure over the injection site. Have the patient ice the affected area for 20 minutes two to three times daily for the first 24–48 hours. A wrist splint can be used for several days. Then begin local heat and gentle stretching exercises several days after the injection. Avoid vigorous exercise or heavy lifting for several days.

When to Perform Follow-Up Injections

Although there are no strict guidelines, a reasonable approach is to reinject in 4–6 weeks if symptoms persist or return. Partial relief of symptoms is an indication for a repeat injection. A total of three injections in a given 12-month period is the accepted standard. Botox into the flexor muscles has been reported to be beneficial if corticosteroid/lidocaine injections do not provide relief. If significant pain relief is not obtained after three injections, consider further imaging studies and possible surgical consultation.

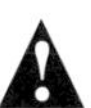

Rotator Cuff Tendinitis

Name of Procedure

This procedure is called injection of the rotator cuff tendons for tendinitis. Although this is commonly referred to as a tendinitis, a more accurate description may be tendinosis because signs of inflammation may be absent. This injection can also help differentiate a rotator cuff tear from a tendinitis because there should be pain relief after injection with tendinitis.

CPT

The Current Procedural Terminology code is 20610 (injection of major joint or bursa) if injection is made in the subacromial bursa 20550 (injection of tendon sheath) if injection is made near insertion of rotator cuff tendons.

Indications

This injection is usually used for rotator cuff tendinitis after a patient has failed a course of NSAID and/or physical therapy. Generally, the tendinitis is in the supraspinatus portion of the rotator cuff.

Symptoms

- Pain in the posterolateral shoulder, more pronounced with overhead activities (especially if the arm is abducted more than 90 degrees).
- Patient may complain of pain with self-care activities, such as combing hair or hooking bras in the back.
- Decreased functional ability secondary to decreased range of motion of the shoulder.

Physical Examination Findings

- Tenderness to palpation of the shoulder.
- Decreased active arm elevation (decreased passive range of motion as well indicates adhesive capsulitis).
- Pain with arm elevation between 60 and 120 degrees.
- Pain with forced shoulder flexion with the humerus internally rotated.
- Positive Dawbarn's sign (pain on palpation over the greater tuberosity of the humerus with the arm hanging down, which is not present when the arm is abducted).
- Weakness of the muscles of the rotator cuff.
- After prolonged periods, muscle wasting or a frozen shoulder may be noted.

Medications to Inject

A corticosteroid and local anesthetic mixture is injected.

Amount to Inject

The injectate amount is 2–3 mL.

Size and Gauge of Needle

A 1–1½-inch 25- to 27-gauge needle is used.

Local Anatomy

The rotator cuff is the musculotendinous unit of four muscles: the supraspinatus, infraspinatus, subscapularis, and teres minor. These muscles help to stabilize the humeral head against the glenoid and rotate the arm. The supraspinatus tendon is most susceptible to injury. The tendons of the musculotendinous junction may become inflamed by impingement on the acromion, the coracoacromial ligament, the acromioclavicular joint, or the coracoid process. The subacromial bursa protects the tendons from the compressive force of the humeral head and the acromion. Poor blood supply to the rotator cuff decreases the ability to heal these structures. If inflammation is continuous, calcium deposition may take place, making treatment more difficult. Tendinitis frequently coexists with bursitis.

Patient Position

The patient is seated with the arm at the side and the hands in the lap.

How and Where to Inject

The injection is generally performed in the subacromial bursa (Figures 4–11 and 4–12). Palpate the acromion and mark its inferolateral margin. Insert the needle in the lateral aspect of the shoulder 1–1½ inches below the middle of the acromion. Direct the needle slightly cephalad. If the humeral head is contacted, withdraw and reinsert in a more superior direction. At approximately 1 inch of insertion, the needle should be in the subacromial bursa. The goal is to bathe the tendon in the medication, not to inject into the tendon. If there is resistance, the needle may be in a ligament or tendon, and the position should be changed. Some physicians prefer to inject near the tendon itself. There should be only slight resistance to injection. If there is resistance, the needle may be in the ligament or tendon, and the position should be changed. Aspirate before injecting to ensure that infection is not present and to avoid intravascular administration.

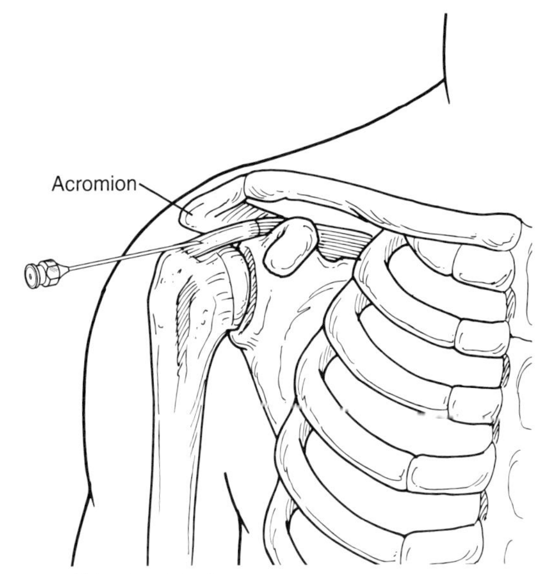

Fig 4–11 Rotator cuff tendon injection.

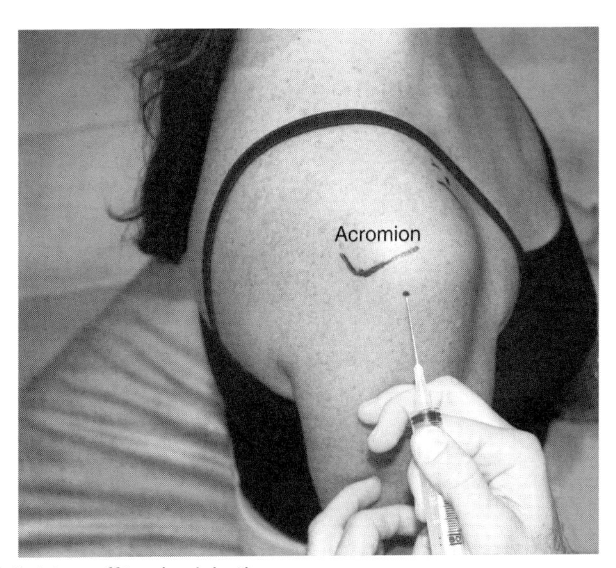

Fig 4–12 Rotator cuff tendon injection.

Pitfalls/Complications

It is anticipated that the patient may have an increase in pain for a few days caused by the use of corticosteroids. Informing patients of this helps to alleviate their postinjection pain concerns. If there is no relief from the injection, consider other sources of pain (rotator cuff tear, bicipital tendinitis, subacromial bursitis, myofascial pain, fracture, adhesive capsulitis, cervical spondylosis, cervical radiculopathy, shoulder arthritis, thoracic outlet syndrome, brachial plexopathy, Pancoast tumor). Occasionally, subcutaneous atrophy and loss of pigmentation can occur. The risk of infection can be minimized with sterile preparation of the area and aseptic technique. Injections directly into the tendon may increase the likelihood of tendon rupture and should be avoided.

Postinjection Care

Apply a sterile dressing and pressure over the injection site. Have the patient ice the affected area for 20 minutes two to three times daily for the first 24–48 hours. Then begin local heat and gentle stretching exercises several days after the injection. Avoid vigorous exercise, heavy lifting, or overhead use of the arm for several days.

When to Perform Follow-Up Injections

Although there are no strict guidelines, a reasonable approach is to reinject in 4–6 weeks if symptoms persist or return. Partial relief of symptoms is an indication for a repeat injection. A total of three injections in a given 12-month period is the accepted standard. If significant pain relief is not obtained after three injections, consider further imaging studies and possible surgical consultation.

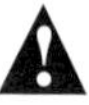

Plantar Fasciitis

Name of Procedure

The term for this procedure is injection of plantar fascia for plantar fasciitis. Although this is commonly referred to as a fasciitis, a more accurate description may be fasciosis because signs of inflammation may be absent.

CPT

The Current Procedural Terminology code is 20605 (injection of intermediate joint or bursa).

Indications

This injection is usually used for plantar fasciitis after a patient has failed a course of NSAID, orthotics (padded arch supports and correction of ankle pronation), taping, Achilles and plantar fascia stretching, and/or physical therapy.

Symptoms

- Pain in the plantar heel.
- Affects women twice as often as men.
- Affects overweight people more than those of normal weight.
- Pain most severe on waking or when rising from a resting position.
- Improved symptoms with nonweightbearing.

Physical Examination Findings

- Pain and tenderness over the medial calcaneal tuberosity and 1–2 cm distally along the plantar fascia.
- May note associated tightness in the Achilles tendon (contributes to increased tension on the plantar fascia).

- Pain with dorsiflexing the toes.

Medications to Inject

A corticosteroid and local anesthetic mixture is injected.

Amount to Inject

The injectate amount is 3–5 mL.

Size and Gauge of Needle

A 1–1½-inch 25-gauge needle is used.

Local Anatomy

The plantar fascia is a thick, multilayered fibrous aponeurosis, which is tightly attached to the plantar skin. The plantar fascia originates at the medial calcaneal tuberosity and then divides into five bands. Each band inserts onto the transverse tarsal ligament, flexor sheath, volar plate, and periosteum of the base of the proximal phalanges.

Patient Position

The patient is placed in the prone position, with the foot hanging off of the examination table.

How and Where to Inject

The medial aspect of the heel is palpated. Insert the needle approximately 2 cm from the plantar surface of the foot, near the anterior tip of the medial calcaneus (Figures 4–13 and 4–14). Advance the needle to the calcaneus, and then withdraw slightly to the periosteum, and inject slowly as the needle is withdrawn. There should be slight resistance to injection. Do not inject into the fat pad to avoid fat pad atrophy. Aspirate before injecting to ensure that infection is not present and to avoid intravascular administration.

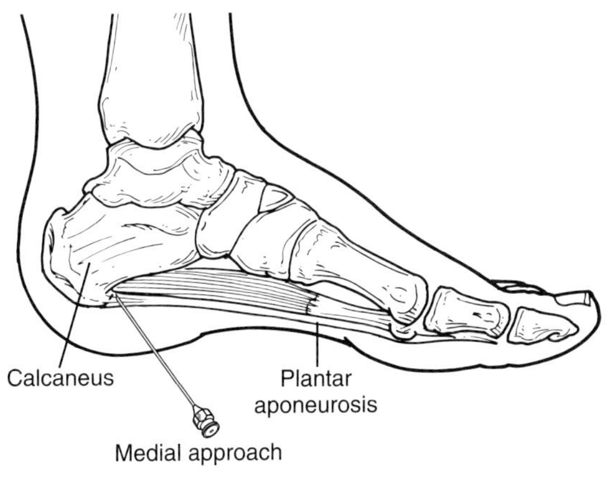

Fig 4–13 Plantar fascia injection.

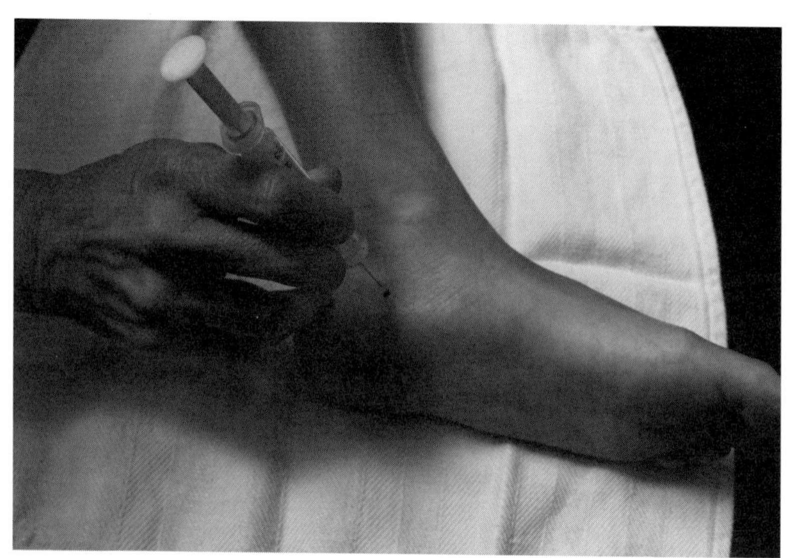

Fig 4–14 Plantar fascia injection.

Pitfalls/Complications

It is anticipated that the patient may have an increase in pain for a few days caused by the use of corticosteroids. Informing patients of this helps to alleviate their postinjection pain concerns. If there is no relief from the injection, consider other sources of pain (tarsal tunnel syndrome, arthritis, gout, occult bony pathology or tumor, rupture of the plantar fascia, sciatic nerve injury, entrapment of the first branch of the lateral plantar nerve). Occasionally, subcutaneous atrophy and loss of pigmentation can occur. Atrophy in the fat pad of the heel could cause gait disturbances. Plantar fascia rupture can occur. The risk of infection can be minimized with sterile preparation of the area and aseptic technique.

Postinjection Care

Apply a sterile dressing and pressure over the injection site. Have the patient ice the affected area for 20 minutes two to three times daily for the first 24–48 hours. Then begin local heat and gentle stretching exercises several days after the injection. Avoid vigorous exercise or running for several days. Passive stretching of the ankle can begin after the pain has resolved. Initiate a physical therapy program, including flexibility training and correction of biomechanical factors. A heel support can be used for the first week after the injection.

When to Perform Follow-Up Injections

Although there are no strict guidelines, a reasonable approach is to reinject in 4–6 weeks if symptoms persist or return. Partial relief of symptoms is an indication for a repeat injection. A total of three injections in a given 12-month period is the accepted standard. If significant pain relief is not obtained after three injections, consider further imaging studies and possible surgical consultation.

Achilles Tendinitis

Name of Procedure

This procedure is termed injection of the Achilles tendon for Achilles tendinitis. Although this is commonly referred to as a tendinitis, a more accurate description may be tendinosis because signs of inflammation may be absent.

CPT

The Current Procedural Terminology code is 20550 (injection of tendon sheath).

Indications

This injection is usually used for Achilles tendinitis after a patient has failed a course of NSAID, counterforce bracing, a heel lift, and/or physical therapy.

Symptoms

- Pain, swelling, and tenderness over the area of the Achilles tendon.
- Usually associated with running sports or a change in the training schedule.
- May be associated with a change in shoe.
- Pain may improve with exercise.

Physical Examination Findings

- Swelling and tenderness to palpation over the Achilles tendon (usually located 5 cm proximal to the calcaneal insertion).
- Decreased range of motion in the ankle.
- Bursitis of the tendon and ankle joint may coexist.
- Pain with resisted plantarflexion.

Medications to Inject

A corticosteroid and local anesthetic mixture is injected.

Amount to Inject

The injectate amount is 1–2 mL.

Size and Gauge of Needle

A 1–1½-inch 25-gauge needle is used.

Local Anatomy

The Achilles tendon begins at mid-calf and inserts in the posterior calcaneus. It narrows towards the insertion, becoming most narrow approximately 5 cm above the calcaneal insertion. A bursa is located between the Achilles tendon and the tibia and calcaneus.

Patient Position

The patient is placed in the prone position with the affected foot slightly dorsiflexed and hanging off the end of the table. Dorsiflexing the foot will help to identify the tendon, which must not be directly injected.

How and Where to Inject

Inject into the area of tenderness (usually located approximately 5 cm proximal to the calcaneal insertion of the tendon) (Figures 4–15 and 4–16). This is a relatively superficial

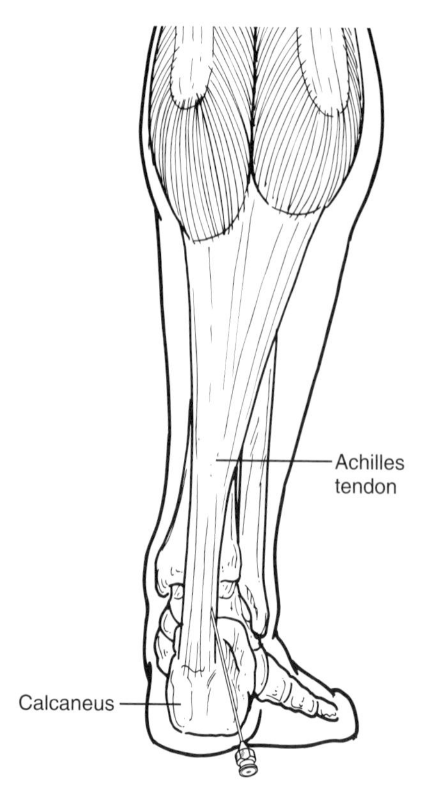

Fig 4–15 Achilles tendon injection.

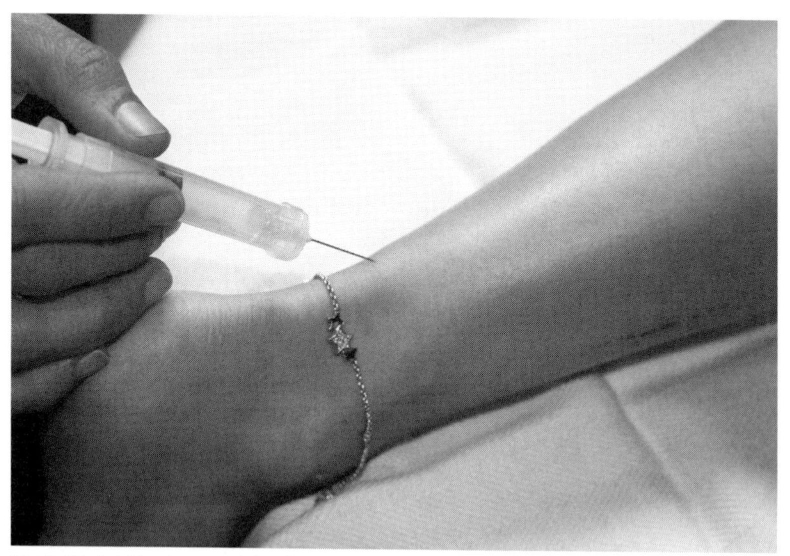

Fig 4–16 Achilles tendon injection.

injection. Once the needle is in, ask the patient to dorsiflex the ankle. If the needle moves with the ankle, you are in the tendon. Pull the needle back 1 mm at a time so that you are in the tendon sheath and not the tendon. If there is resistance, the needle may be in a ligament or tendon, and the position should be changed.

Pitfalls/Complications

It is anticipated that the patient may have an increase in pain for a few days caused by the use of corticosteroids. Informing patients of this helps to alleviate their postinjection pain concerns. If there is no relief from the injection, consider other sources of pain (partial or complete rupture of the Achilles tendon, tibia stress fracture, bursitis, tear in the gastrocnemius muscle, Haglund's syndrome, which is enlargement of the posterosuperior tuberosity of the calcaneus). Because this is a superficial injection, occasionally subcutaneous atrophy and loss of pigmentation can occur. The risk of infection can be minimized with sterile preparation of the area and aseptic technique. Injections directly into the tendon may increase the likelihood of tendon rupture and should be avoided. Aspirate before injecting to avoid intravascular administration.

Postinjection Care

Apply a sterile dressing and pressure over the injection site. Have the patient ice the affected area for 20 minutes two to three times daily for the first 24–48 hours. Then begin local heat and gentle stretching exercises several days after the injection. Avoid vigorous exercise or running for several weeks. Initiate a physical therapy program. Instruct the patient in the importance of stretching the gastrocnemius and soleus muscles and Achilles tendon before exercise.

When to Perform Follow-Up Injections

Although there are no strict guidelines, a reasonable approach is to reinject in 4–6 weeks if symptoms persist or return. Partial relief of symptoms is an indication for a repeat injection. A total of three injections in a given 12-month period is the accepted standard. If significant pain relief is not obtained after three injections, consider further imaging studies and possible surgical consultation.

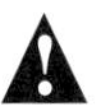

Iliotibial Band Tendinitis/Bursitis

Name of Procedure

This procedure is termed injection of the iliotibial band for iliotibial band tendinitis or bursitis. Although this is often referred to as a tendinitis, the iliotibial band is actually composed of fascia. A more common term is iliotibial band syndrome. The pain is usually attributable to friction as the iliotibial band impinges over the lateral femoral epicondyle.

CPT

The Current Procedural Terminology code is 20610 (injection of major bursa).

Indications

This injection is usually used for iliotibial band tendinitis/bursitis after a patient has failed a course of NSAID, decreasing or modifying athletic activities that exacerbate the pain, addressing the biomechanical causes of pain, and/or physical therapy.

Symptoms

- Lateral knee and/or hip pain.
- Pain aggravated during repetitive activities.
- Patient may complain of "snapping" of the iliotibial band as it passes the greater trochanter.

Physical Examination Findings

- Pain worse with 20–30 degrees of knee flexion.
- Tenderness to palpation at the lateral femoral condyle.
- Iliotibial band swelling may be present.

Medications to Inject

A corticosteroid and local anesthetic mixture is injected.

Amount to Inject

The injectate amount is 2–4 mL.

Size and Gauge of Needle

A 1–1½-inch 25-gauge needle is used.

Local Anatomy

The iliotibial band is a dense fascia on the lateral aspect of the knee and hip that has origins from the gluteus maximus, gluteus medius, and tensor fascia lata muscles. The iliotibial band has aponeurotic connections to the patella and the vastus lateralis. Tendinitis of the iliotibial band may coexist with iliotibial bursitis. There is a "pouch" underlying the posterior iliotibial band at the level of the lateral femoral condyle.

Patient Position

The patient lies in the supine position with a towel underneath the knee so that the knee is slightly flexed.

How and Where to Inject

Injections should be directed to the point of maximum tenderness along the iliotibial band (Figures 4–17 and 4–18). Often, this is into the anatomical pouch at the lateral femoral condyle. Some clinicians will advance the needle to the bone and then withdraw slightly. There should be little resistance to injection. Aspirate before injecting to ensure that infection is not present and to avoid intravascular administration.

Pitfalls/Complications

It is anticipated that the patient may have an increase in pain for a few days caused by the use of corticosteroids. Informing patients of this helps to alleviate their postinjection pain concerns. If there is no relief from the injection, consider other sources of pain (lateral meniscal injury, trochanteric bursitis, hip or knee joint pathology, arthritis, lateral collateral ligamentous injury, lateral hamstring tear). Occasionally, subcutaneous atrophy and loss of pigmentation can occur. The risk of infection can be minimized with sterile preparation of the area and aseptic technique. Injections directly into the tendon may increase the likelihood of tendon rupture and should be avoided.

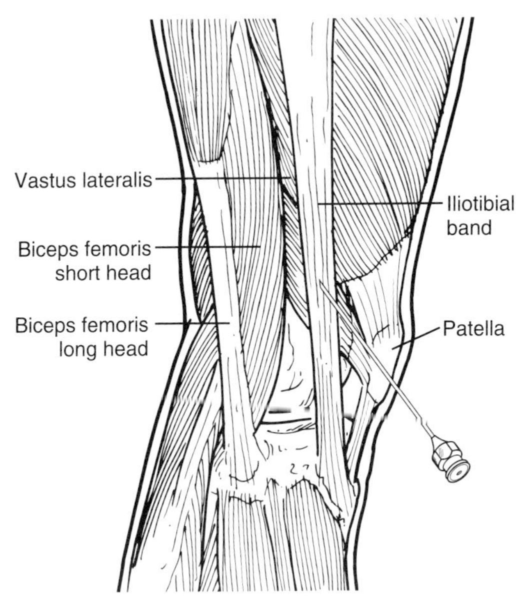

Fig 4–17 Iliotibial band injection.

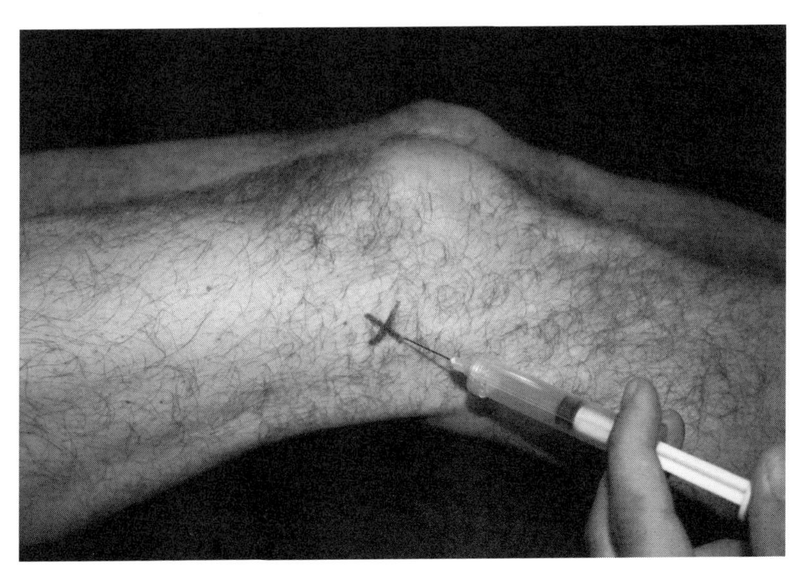

Fig 4–18 Iliotibial band injection.

Postinjection Care

Apply pressure over the injection site. Have the patient ice the affected area for 20 minutes two to three times daily for the first 24–48 hours. Then begin local heat and gentle stretching exercises several days after the injection. Avoid vigorous exercise or running for several days. A strengthening and stretching program of the gluteus medius and tensor fascia lata should be started after a week. Because footwear and running technique can contribute to the development of this condition, they should be evaluated.

When to Perform Follow-Up Injections

Although there are no strict guidelines, a reasonable approach is to reinject in 4–6 weeks if symptoms persist or return. Partial relief of symptoms is an indication for a repeat injection. A total of three injections in a given 12-month period is the accepted standard. If significant pain relief is not obtained after three injections, consider further imaging studies.

Infrapatellar Tendinitis

Name of Procedure

This procedure is termed injection of the infrapatellar tendon for infrapatellar tendinitis. Although this is commonly referred to as a tendinitis, a more accurate description may be tendinosis because signs of inflammation may be absent.

CPT

The Current Procedural Terminology code is 20051 (injection of tendon).

Indications

This injection is usually used for infrapatellar tendinitis after a patient has failed a course of NSAID, decreasing or modifying athletic activities that exacerbate the pain, knee immobilization, addressing the biomechanical causes of pain, and/or physical therapy. Some physicians do not advocate injection at all, whereas others find it helpful if conservative management has failed.

Symptoms

- Anterior knee pain (patient may be able to point to a tender point along the tibial tubercle).
- Pain aggravated by sitting, squatting, climbing stairs, or kneeling.

Physical Examination Findings

- Pain worse with resisted extension or passive hyperflexion of the knee.
- Tenderness to palpation at the point where the tendon inserts on the tibial tubercle.
- Swelling may be present.
- May see quadriceps atrophy with long-standing condition.

Medications to Inject

A corticosteroid and local anesthetic mixture is injected.

Amount to Inject

The injectate amount is 2–4 mL.

Size and Gauge of Needle

A 1–1½-inch 25-gauge needle is used.

Local Anatomy

The infrapatellar tendon originates at the inferior pole of the patella and inserts at the tibial tubercle.

Patient Position

The patient lies in the supine position with a towel underneath the knee so that the knee is slightly flexed.

How and Where to Inject

Injections should be directed to the point of maximum tenderness (Figures 4–19 and 4–20). Some clinicians will advance the needle to the bone and then withdraw slightly. There should be little resistance to injection. If resistance is met, the needle may be in the tendon. Withdraw the needle until no resistance is met. The goal is to inject around the tendon, not into the tendon, because injecting into the tendon increases the likelihood of

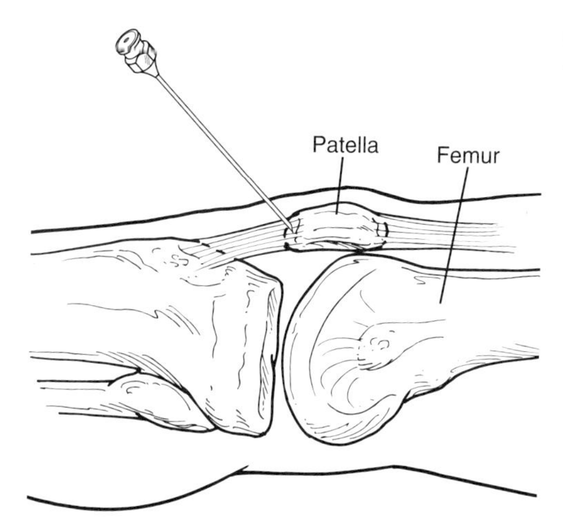

Fig 4–19 Infrapatellar tendon injection.

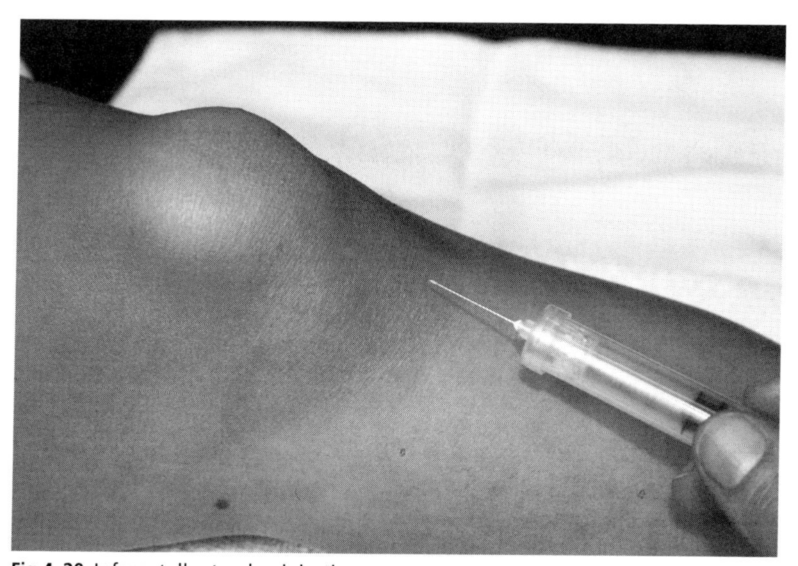

Fig 4–20 Infrapatellar tendon injection.

tendon rupture. Aspirate before injecting to ensure that infection is not present and to avoid intravascular administration.

Pitfalls/Complications

It is anticipated that the patient may have an increase in pain for a few days caused by the use of corticosteroids. Informing patients of this helps to alleviate their postinjection pain concerns. If there is no relief from the injection, consider other sources of pain (tendon rupture, anterior or posterior cruciate ligament injury, infrapatellar bursitis, meniscal injuries, chondromalacia patella, infection). Occasionally, subcutaneous atrophy and loss of pigmentation can occur. The risk of infection can be minimized with sterile preparation of the area and aseptic technique. Injections directly into the tendon may increase the likelihood of tendon rupture and should be avoided.

Postinjection Care

Apply a sterile dressing and pressure over the injection site. Have the patient ice the affected area for 20 minutes two to three times daily for the first 24–48 hours. Then begin local heat and gentle stretching exercises several days after the injection. Avoid vigorous exercise or running for several days. A period of relative rest should follow, avoiding all activities that exacerbated the pain.

When to Perform Follow-Up Injections

Although there are no strict guidelines, a reasonable approach is to reinject in 4–6 weeks if symptoms persist or return. Partial relief of symptoms is an indication for a repeat injection. A total of three injections in a given 12-month period is the accepted standard. If significant pain relief is not obtained after three injections, consider further imaging studies.

5

Bursae

The injection procedures here are based on a review of the various techniques described in the medical literature as well as the authors' experiences. The techniques chosen are felt to be the most appropriate in most cases. As clinical circumstances may differ, other approaches may be more appropriate for individual cases. The reader is encouraged to familiarize himself/herself with the additional sources in the bibliography at the end of this chapter for additional approaches.

All procedures should be performed using appropriate preparation and aseptic technique. Local anesthesia (either injected or vapo-coolant spray) may be helpful in most procedures. As always, the clinician should weigh the risks and benefits of any interventional procedure.

Subacromial Bursa (Subdeltoid Bursa)

Name of Procedure

The procedure is called a subacromial bursa (subdeltoid bursa) injection.

CPT

The Current Procedural Terminology code is 20610 (injection of major joint or bursa).

Indications

Subacromial bursitis (sometimes referred to as subdeltoid bursitis) is the indication for subacromial bursa injection. This can be a first-line treatment for subacromial bursitis, or it can be a treatment offered after a patient has had a course of NSAIDs and/or physical therapy (including weighted pendulum exercises). Some physicians use injections of the subacromial bursa for diagnostic as well as therapeutic reasons. A diagnosis of shoulder impingement, supraspinatus tendinitis, or subacromial (subdeltoid) bursitis is suggested after a reduction of pain.

Symptoms

- Anterior and lateral shoulder pain.
- Difficulty sleeping on affected side.
- Pain with shoulder abduction.

Physical Examination Findings

- Pain with direct palpation over the subacromial bursa.
- Limited active and passive shoulder abduction.
- Positive impingement sign.

Medications to Inject

A corticosteroid and local anesthetic mixture is injected.

Amount to Inject

The injectate amount is approximately 5 mL.

Size and Gauge of Needle

A 1¼–1½-inch 22- to 25-gauge needle is used—the length of the needle will depend on how much subcutaneous tissue is in the affected area.

Local Anatomy

The subacromial bursa lies on the supraspinatus tendon and is covered by the acromion, the coracoacromial ligament, and the deltoid. Inflammation of the rotator cuff tendons frequently coexists with the bursitis.

Patient Position

The patient is seated with the arm at the side and the hands resting on the lap.

How and Where to Inject

Palpate the acromion and mark its inferolateral margin (Figures 5–1 and 5–2). Insert the needle in the lateral aspect of the shoulder 1–1½ inches below the middle of the acromion. Direct the needle slightly cephalad. If the humeral head is contacted, withdraw and reinsert in a more superior direction. At approximately 1 inch deep, the needle should be in the subacromial bursa. The goal is to inject into the bursa, not to inject into the tendon. If there is resistance, the needle may be in a ligament or tendon, and the position should be changed. Some physicians prefer to inject near the tendon itself. If the aim of the injection is to approximate the supraspinatus tendon, the needle is positioned over the anterior edge of the acromion. Direct the needle perpendicularly until the bone is reached. Withdraw the needle 1–2 mm and inject. There should be only slight resistance to injection. If there is resistance, the needle may be in the ligament or tendon, and the position

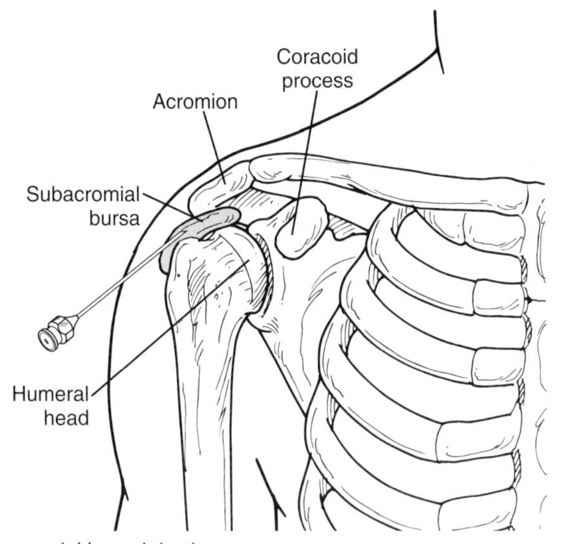

Fig 5–1 Subacromial bursa injection.

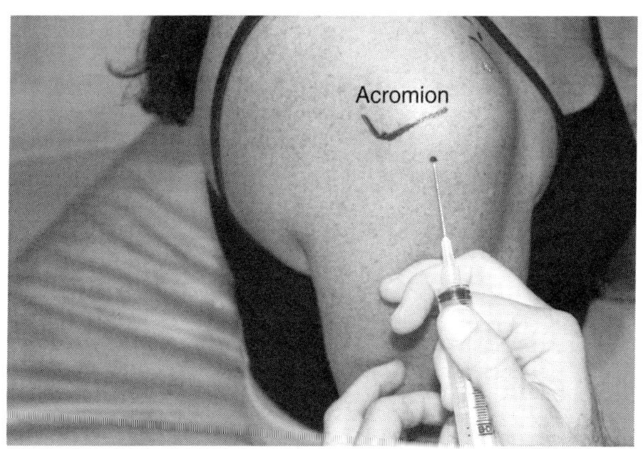

Fig 5–2 Subacromial bursa injection.

should be changed. Aspirate before injecting to ensure that infection is not present and to avoid intravascular administration.

Pitfalls/Complications

It is anticipated that the patient may have an increase in pain for a few days caused by the use of corticosteroids. Informing patients of this helps to alleviate their postinjection pain concerns. If there is no relief from the injection, consider other sources of pain (rotator cuff tendinitis, rotator cuff tear, arthritis, cervical disk disorder). Also, consider whether the medication actually reached the subacromial bursa. The risk of infection can be minimized with sterile preparation of the area and aseptic technique.

Postinjection Care

Apply a sterile dressing and pressure over the injection site. Have the patient ice the affected area for 20 minutes two to three times daily for the first 24–48 hours. Then begin local heat and gentle stretching exercises several days after the injection. Avoid vigorous exercise or overhead activities for several days.

When to Perform Follow-Up Injections

Although there are no strict guidelines, a reasonable approach is to reinject in 4–6 weeks if symptoms persist or return. Partial relief of symptoms is an indication for a repeat injection. A total of three injections in a given 12-month period is the accepted standard. If significant pain relief is not obtained after three injections, consider further imaging studies.

Olecranon Bursa

Name of Procedure

The name of this procedure is injection of the olecranon bursa.

CPT

The Current Procedural Terminology code is 20605 (injection of intermediate joint or bursa).

Indications

The indication for this injection is olecranon bursitis. Aspiration is often considered a first-line treatment. After aspiration, injection of the bursa can be performed. Some physicians will inject after a patient has had a course of NSAID and/or physical therapy.

Symptoms

- A swelling may be noted over the bursa at the elbow.
- Pain at the site of the bursa (usually indicates infectious or traumatic origin).

Physical Examination Findings

- A large mass may be palpable over the tip of the elbow.
- The area may be erythematous and tender (tenderness usually indicates infectious or traumatic origin).
- With chronic inflammation, calcification of the bursa may occur, resulting in a sensation of touching gravel when palpating the bursa.
- Reproduction of pain with passive elbow extension.

Medications to Inject

A corticosteroid and local anesthetic mixture is injected.

Amount to Inject

The injectate amount is 2–4 mL.

Size and Gauge of Needle

A 1½-inch 18- to 20-gauge needle is used to aspirate, and a 1½-inch 22- to 25-gauge needle is used to inject.

Local Anatomy

The olecranon bursa lies between the skin and the olecranon process of the ulna at the elbow. Because of its subcutaneous position, it is susceptible to injury. The ulnar nerve lies in the ulnar groove between the medial epicondyle and the olecranon of the ulna.

Patient Position

The patient is positioned supine with the affected arm adducted and the elbow flexed. The patient's palm should rest on the abdomen.

How and Where to Inject

Insert the needle into the swollen area overlying the olecranon (Figures 5–3 and 5–4). Avoid inserting medial to the olecranon to avoid injuring the ulnar nerve. The bursa is relatively superficial. Aspirate the bursa before injecting. (This may often require multiple changes in the needle trajectory during aspiration because the swollen bursa are often multiloculated.) If the aspirate appears positive for infection (cloudy), do not inject. Bursal fluid should undergo microscopic examination for crystals (gout), cell count, Gram stain, and culture. If blood is aspirated, the diagnosis may be hemorrhagic bursitis. Aspiration, but not injection, should be performed under these circumstances. If injecting, inject perpendicular to the swelling, keeping the bevel of the needle facing the bone. If the needle hits the bone, the needle is withdrawn slightly into the bursa. There should be little resistance to injection if the needle is in the bursa. If there is resistance, the needle may be in a ligament or tendon, and the position should be changed. Aspirate before injecting to ensure that infection is not present and to avoid intravascular administration.

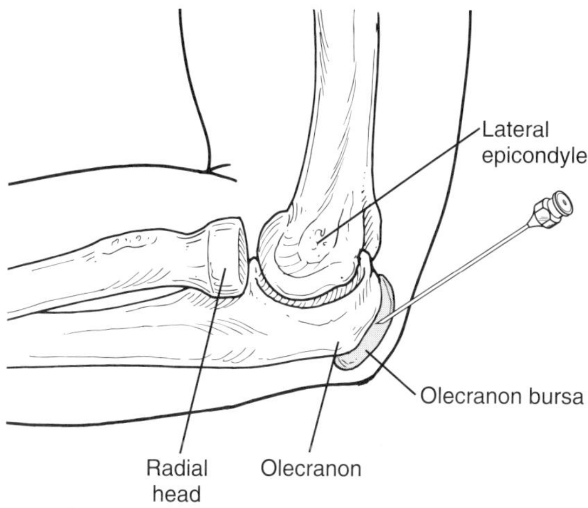

Fig 5–3 Olecranon bursa injection.

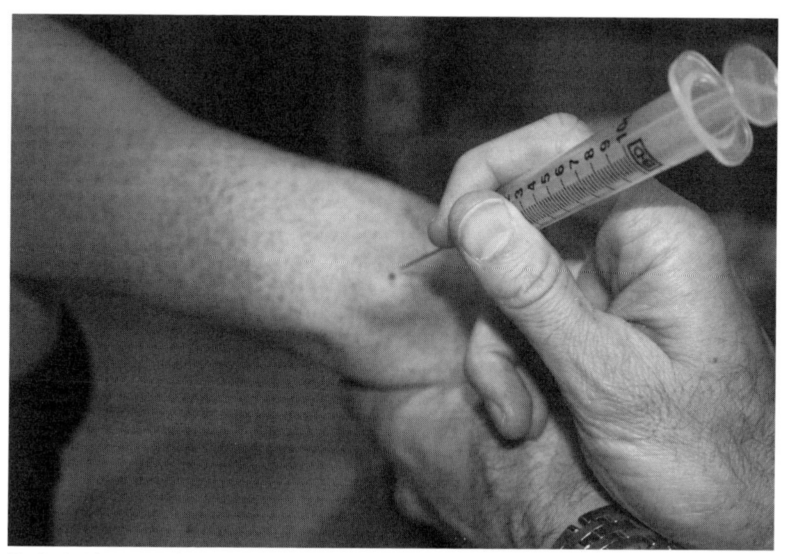

Fig 5–4 Olecranon bursa injection.

Pitfalls/Complications

It is anticipated that the patient may have an increase in pain for a few days caused by the use of corticosteroids. Informing patients of this helps to alleviate their postinjection pain concerns. If there is no relief from the injection, consider other sources of pain (fracture of the olecranon process, rheumatoid arthritis, gout, infection, chondrocalcinosis, lipoma, hemorrhagic bursitis). Also, consider whether the medication actually reached the olecranon bursa. The risk of infection can be minimized with sterile preparation of the area and aseptic technique. Tendon rupture can occur if corticosteroids are injected directly into a tendon. Avoid the ulnar nerve by injecting into the lateral aspect of the bursa. Because this is a relatively superficial injection, skin discoloration and subcutaneous atrophy can occur, and the patient should be aware of this possibility.

Postinjection Care

Apply a sterile dressing and pressure over the injection site. Have the patient ice the affected area for 20 minutes two to three times daily for the first 24–48 hours. Then begin local heat and gentle stretching exercises several days after the injection. Avoid vigorous exercise or use of the arm for several days. Consider the use of an elbow pad to protect the area.

When to Perform Follow-Up Injections

Although there are no strict guidelines, a reasonable approach is to reinject in 4–6 weeks if symptoms persist or return. Partial relief of symptoms is an indication for a repeat injection. A total of three injections in a given 12-month period is the accepted standard. If significant pain relief is not obtained after three injections, consider further imaging studies.

Trochanteric Bursa

Name of Procedure

The name of this procedure is trochanteric bursa injection.

CPT

The Current Procedural Terminology code is 20610 (injection of major joint or bursa).

Indication

The indication for this injection is trochanteric bursitis. This can be a first-line treatment for trochanteric bursitis, or it can be a treatment offered after a patient has had a course of NSAIDs and/or physical therapy.

Symptoms

- Pain in lateral aspect of the thigh, especially during ambulation.
- Pain may mimic sciatica.
- Pain while lying on the affected side.
- Pain with walking up stairs.
- Symptoms after trauma (fall) or overuse (running on soft or uneven surfaces).
- May be associated with iliotibial band tendinitis.

Physical Examination Findings

- Pain with direct palpation to the trochanteric bursa.
- Reproduction of pain with the leg in external rotation and abduction.

Medications to Inject

A corticosteroid and local anesthetic mixture is injected.

Amount to Inject

The injectate amount is 2–5 mL.

Size and Gauge of Needle

A 1.5–3.5-inch 22- to 25-gauge needle is used. The length of the needle will depend on how much subcutaneous tissue is in the affected area. People who have more adipose tissue will require the use of a longer needle.

Local Anatomy

The trochanteric bursa lies between the greater trochanter and the tendon of the gluteus medius and the iliotibial tract.

Patient Position

The patient is in the lateral decubitus position with the knees flexed to 90 degrees.

How and Where to Inject

Direct the needle to the point of maximal tenderness over the greater trochanter (Figures 5–5 and 5–6). Direct the needle through the gluteus medius tendon/iliotibial band, and then inject directly into the bursa, which lies in close proximity to the bone. Many clinicians find it helpful to locate the bursa by going all the way to the bone and then pulling back approximately ¼ inch. There should be little resistance to injection if the needle is in the bursa. Aspirate before injecting to ensure that infection is not present and to avoid intravascular administration.

Pitfalls/Complications

It is anticipated that the patient may have an increase in pain for a few days caused by the use of corticosteroids. Informing patients of this helps to alleviate their postinjection pain concerns. If there is no relief from the injection, consider other sources of pain (spine, hip or knee arthritis, scoliosis, tumor, leg length discrepancy, iliotibial band tightness, avascular necrosis of the femoral head, lumbar radiculopathy, trochanteric fracture, meralgia paresthetica). Also, consider whether the medication actually reached the trochanteric bursa. The risk of infection can be minimized with sterile preparation of the area and aseptic technique.

Postinjection Care

Apply a sterile dressing and pressure over the injection site. Have the patient ice the affected area for 20 minutes two to three times daily for the first 24–48 hours. Then begin

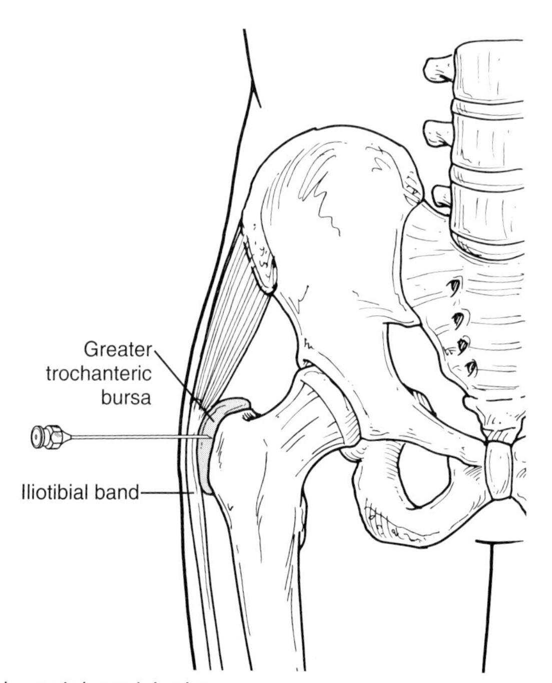

Fig 5–5 Trochanteric bursa injection.

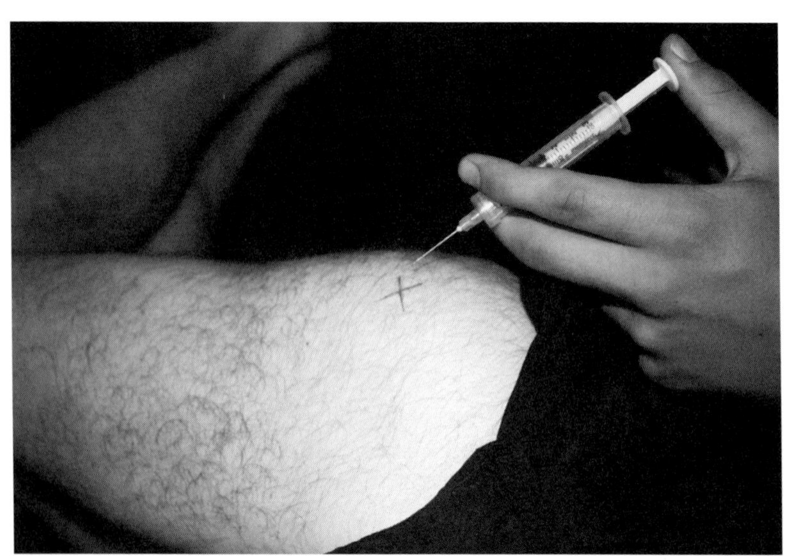

Fig 5–6 Trochanteric bursa injection.

local heat and gentle stretching exercises several days after the injection. Avoid vigorous exercise, repetitive bending, or running for several days. Cross-leg stretching exercises of the gluteus medius muscle may begin after pain has subsided.

When to Perform Follow-Up Injections

Although there are no strict guidelines, a reasonable approach is to reinject in 4–6 weeks if symptoms persist or return. Partial relief of symptoms is an indication for a repeat injection. A total of three injections in a given 12-month period is the accepted standard. If significant pain relief is not obtained after three injections, consider further imaging studies.

Ischial Bursa

Name of Procedure

This procedure is called an ischial bursa injection.

CPT

The Current Procedural Terminology code is 20610 (injection of major joint or bursa).

Indications

The indication for this injection is ischial bursitis. This can be a first-line treatment for ischial bursitis, or it can be a treatment offered after a patient has had a course of NSAIDs and/or physical therapy.

Symptoms

- Pain while sitting.
- Pain with walking up stairs or up hills.
- Symptoms after trauma (fall) or overuse (running on soft or uneven surfaces).

Physical Examination Findings

- Pain with direct palpation to the ischial bursa.
- Pain with resisted leg extension or passive straight-leg raising.

Medications to Inject

A corticosteroid and local anesthetic mixture is injected.

Amount to Inject

The injectate amount is 5 mL.

Size and Gauge of Needle

A 3–3.5 inch 22 gauge needle is used—the length of the needle will depend on how much subcutaneous tissue is in the affected area. Patients who have more adipose tissue will require the use of a longer needle.

Local Anatomy

The ischial bursa lies between the ischial tuberosity and the gluteus maximus muscle. The sciatic nerve is located lateral to the bursa.

Patient Position

The patient lies on the unaffected side with the knees fully flexed.

How and Where to Inject

Palpate the ischial tuberosity. This should correspond with the area of maximal tenderness if the ischial bursa is the origin of pain (Figures 5–7 and 5–8). Direct the needle to the point of maximal tenderness over the ischial tuberosity. Inject directly into the bursa, which lies in close proximity to the bone. Many clinicians find it helpful to locate the bursa by going all the way to the bone and then withdrawing slightly into the bursa. If the patient experiences paresthesias, the needle may be touching the sciatic nerve. Reposition the needle medially. There should be little resistance to injection if the needle is in the bursa. If there is resistance, the needle may be in a ligament or tendon, and the position should be changed. Aspirate before injecting to ensure that infection is not present and to avoid intravascular administration.

Pitfalls/Complications

It is anticipated that the patient may have an increase in pain for a few days caused by the use of corticosteroids. Informing patients of this helps to alleviate their postinjection pain concerns. If there is no relief from the injection, consider other sources of pain (ischial apophysitis, hamstring tendinitis). Also, consider whether the medication actually reached the ischial bursa. The risk of infection can be minimized with sterile preparation of the area and aseptic technique.

Postinjection Care

Apply a sterile dressing and pressure over the injection site. Have the patient ice the affected area for 20 minutes two to three times daily for the first 24–48 hours. Then begin local heat and gentle stretching exercises several days after the injection. Avoid vigorous exercise or running for several days.

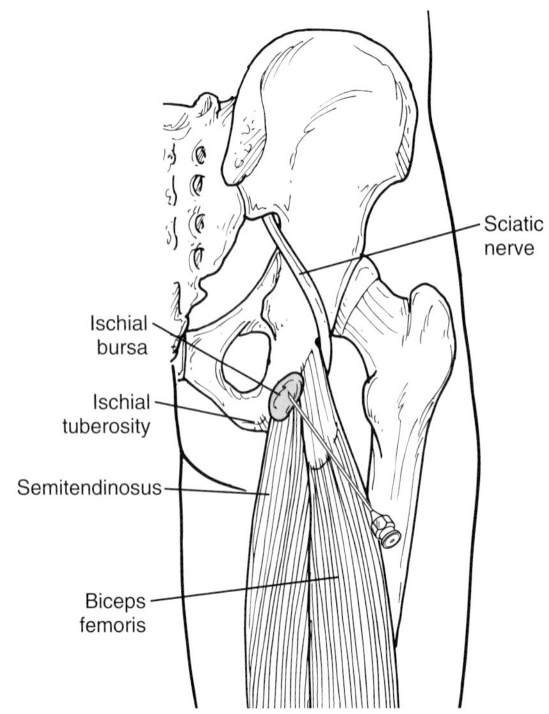

Fig 5–7 Ischial bursa injection.

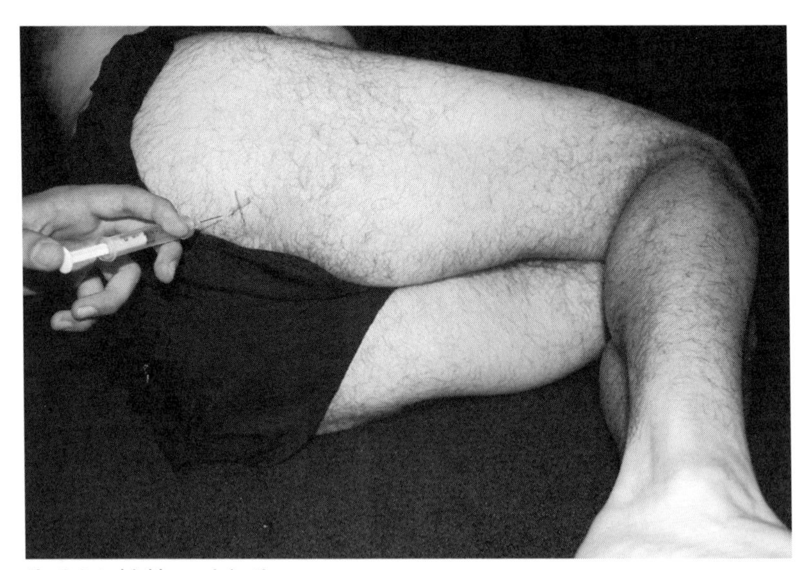

Fig 5–8 Ischial bursa injection.

When to Perform Follow-Up Injections

Although there are no strict guidelines, a reasonable approach is to reinject in 4–6 weeks if symptoms persist or return. Partial relief of symptoms is an indication for a repeat injection. A total of three injections in a given 12-month period is the accepted standard. If significant pain relief is not obtained after three injections, consider further imaging studies.

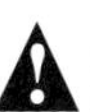

Pes Anserine Bursa

Name of Procedure

The name of this procedure is injection of pes anserine bursa.

CPT

The Current Procedural Terminology code is 20610 (injection of major joint or bursa)

Indications

The indication for this injection is pes anserine bursitis. This can be a first-line treatment for pes anserine bursitis, or it can be a treatment offered after a patient has had a course of NSAID and/or physical therapy (including attempts at correcting gait disturbances).

Symptoms

- Pain over the medial knee joint.
- Pain with activity involving knee flexion and external rotation.
- Pain with kneeling or walking up steps.
- Commonly seen in overweight women with osteoarthritis of the knee.
- May be associated with pes planus.

Physical Examination Findings

- Tenderness to palpation over the bursa (anteromedial knee just distal to the medial knee joint at the tendinous insertion of the pes anserine tendon).
- Increased pain with knee flexion.
- Increased pain with passive valgus stretch of the knee.
- Increased pain with active resisted flexion of the knee.
- May see swelling of the bursa.

Medications to Inject

A corticosteroid and local anesthetic mixture is injected.

Amount to Inject

The injectate amount is 1–3 mL.

Size and Gauge of Needle

A 1½-inch 22- to 25-gauge needle is used.

Local Anatomy

The pes anserine bursa lies beneath the pes anserine tendon (composed of the insertional tendon of the sartorius, gracilis, and semitendinosus muscles). It is located on the medial side of the tibia. The pes anserine tendons cross the medial collateral ligament.

Patient Position

The patient is in the supine position with a towel under the knee so that the knee joint is slightly flexed and the leg is externally rotated.

How and Where to Inject

Point tenderness should be noted in a spot approximately 1½ inches distal to the medial joint space (parallel to the tibial tubercle) where the pes anserine tendon attaches to the tibia (Figures 5–9 and 5–10). The needle is inserted at a 45-degree angle to the tibia. It is inserted through the tendon to the bursa. If the needle hits the bone, the needle is withdrawn slightly into the bursa. There should be little resistance to injection if the needle is in the bursa. If there is resistance, the needle may be in the medial collateral ligament or the tendon, and the position should be changed. Aspirate before injecting to ensure that infection is not present and to avoid intravascular administration.

Pitfalls/Complications

It is anticipated that the patient may have an increase in pain for a few days caused by the use of corticosteroids. Informing patients of this helps to alleviate their postinjection pain concerns. If there is no relief from the injection, consider other sources of pain (tendinitis, bursitis in the knee but not at the pes anserine bursa, medial meniscal tear, arthritis, saphenous nerve entrapment, internal derangement of the knee, especially the medial collateral ligament). Also, consider whether the medication actually reached the pes anserine bursa. The risk of infection can be minimized with sterile preparation of the area and aseptic technique. Tendon rupture can occur if corticosteroids are injected directly into the tendon.

Postinjection Care

Apply a sterile dressing and pressure over the injection site. Have the patient ice the affected area for 20 minutes two to three times daily for the first 24–48 hours. Then begin

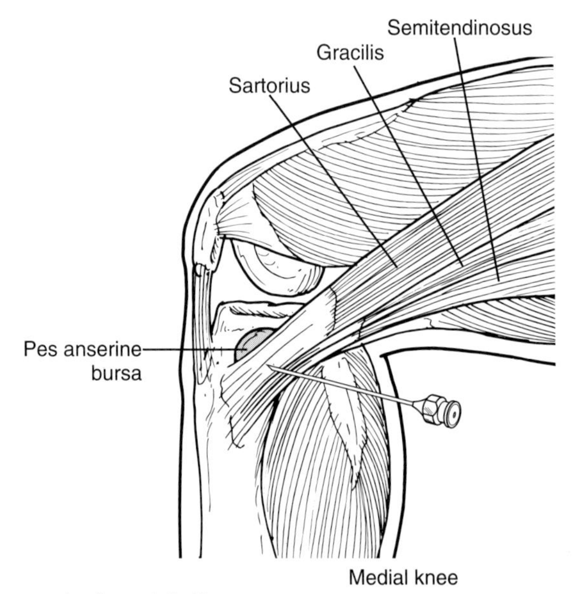

Fig 5–9 Pes anserine bursa injection.

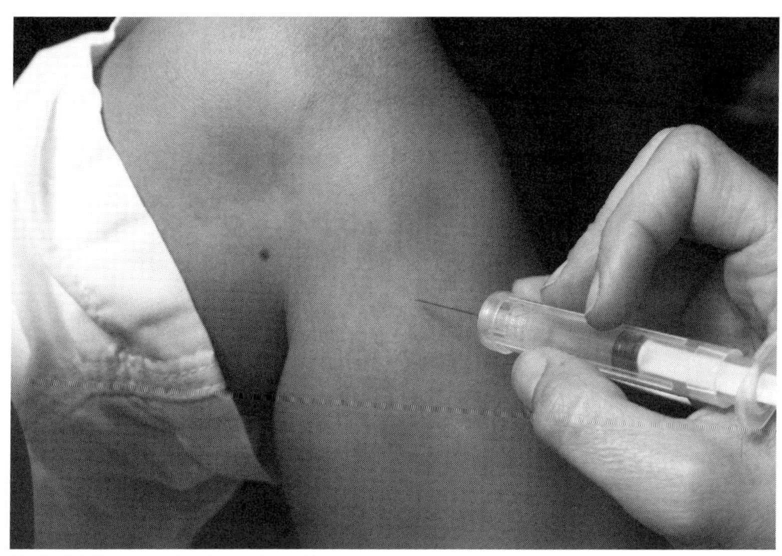

Fig 5–10 Pes anserine bursa injection.

local heat and gentle stretching exercises several days after the injection. Avoid vigorous exercise or running for several days.

When to Perform Follow-Up Injections

Although there are no strict guidelines, a reasonable approach is to reinject in 4–6 weeks if symptoms persist or return. Partial relief of symptoms is an indication for a repeat injection. A total of up to three injections in a given 12-month period is the accepted standard. If significant pain relief is not obtained after three injections, consider further imaging studies.

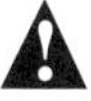

Prepatellar Bursa

Name of Procedure

This procedure is called injection of the prepatellar bursa.

CPT

The Current Procedural Terminology code is 20610 (injection of major joint or bursa).

Indications

The indication for this injection is prepatellar bursitis. This can be a firstline treatment for prepatellar bursitis, or it can be a treatment offered after a patient has had a course of NSAID and/or physical therapy (including use of a protective kneepad). This is also referred to as housemaid's knee because it is frequently seen in patients who kneel excessively.

Symptoms

- Swelling over the anterior knee.
- Pain with direct pressure over the knee (i.e., with kneeling).

- Pain with activity involving knee flexion.
- Pain walking down stairs.

Physical Examination Findings

- Tenderness to palpation over the bursa.
- Increased pain with passive knee flexion or resisted knee extension.
- Swelling of the bursa.
- Look for signs of bursa infection (heat, erythema, systemic symptoms).

Medications to Inject

A corticosteroid and local anesthetic mixture is injected.

Amount to Inject

The injectate amount is 1–3 mL.

Size and Gauge of Needle

A 18- to 20-gauge needle is used for aspirating, and a 1½-inch 22- to 25-gauge needle is used for injecting.

Local Anatomy

The prepatellar bursa lies between the patella and the overlying skin.

Patient Position

The patient is in the supine position with the knee extended.

How and Where to Inject

The needle is inserted parallel to the patella into the bursal sac at the middle to superior pole of the patella (Figures 5–11 and 5–12). If the needle hits the bone, the needle is withdrawn slightly into the bursa. This bursa can become infected or inflamed by urate crystals. As such, most physicians prefer to aspirate before injecting. If the aspirate

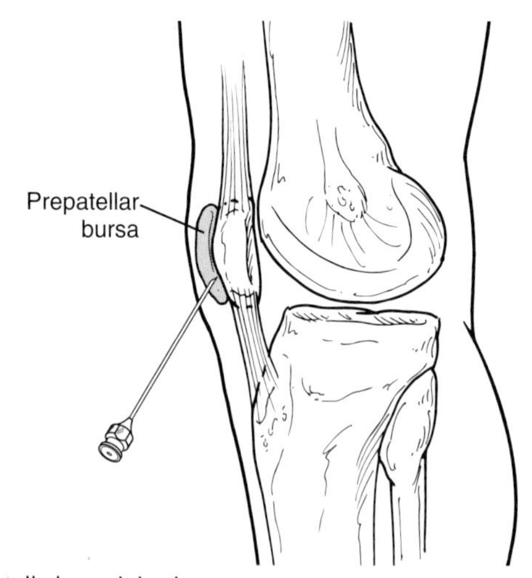

Fig 5–11 Prepatella bursa injection.

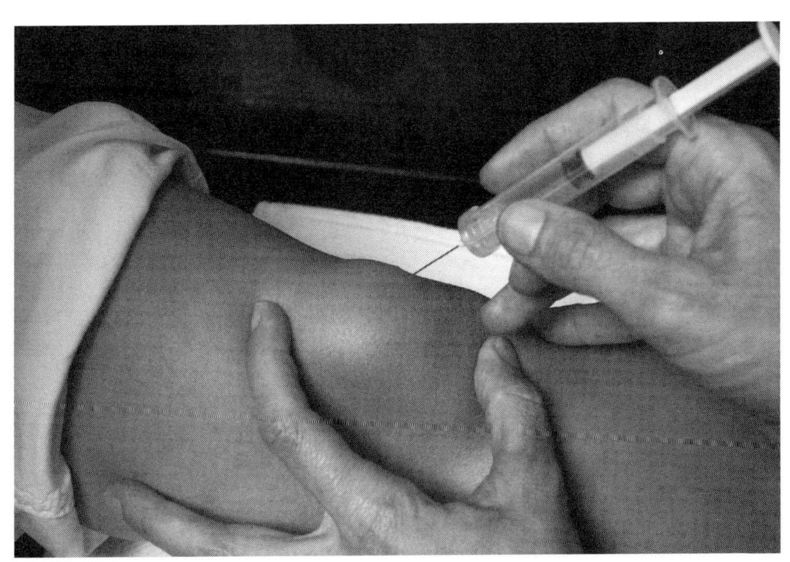

Fig 5–12 Prepatella bursa injection.

appears positive for infection, do not inject. Bursal fluid should undergo microscopic examination for crystals (gout), cell count, Gram stain, and culture. There should be little resistance to injection if the needle is in the bursa. If there is resistance, the needle may be in the tendon or ligament, and the position should be changed. Because the bursa is often multiloculated, repeat injections may be required. Aspirate before injecting to ensure that infection is not present and to avoid intravascular administration.

Pitfalls/Complications

It is anticipated that the patient may have an increase in pain for a few days caused by the use of corticosteroids. Informing patients of this helps to alleviate their postinjection pain concerns. If there is no relief from the injection, consider other sources of pain (patellofemoral subluxation, patellofemoral syndrome, patellar dislocation, quadriceps tendinitis, pes anserine bursitis, meniscal tear, arthritis, femoral nerve entrapment, internal derangement of the knee). Also, consider whether the medication actually reached the bursa. The risk of infection can be minimized with sterile preparation of the area and aseptic technique. Tendon rupture can occur if corticosteroids are injected directly into the tendon. Prepatellar bursitis often coexists with arthritis and tendinitis.

Postinjection Care

Apply a sterile dressing and pressure over the injection site. Have the patient ice the affected area for 20 minutes two to three times daily for the first 24–48 hours. Then begin local heat and gentle stretching exercises several days after the injection. Avoid vigorous exercise or running for several days.

When to Perform Follow-Up Injections

Although there are no strict guidelines, a reasonable approach is to reinject in 4–6 weeks if symptoms persist or return. Partial relief of symptoms is an indication for a repeat injection. A total of up to three injections in a given 12-month period is the accepted standard. If significant pain relief is not obtained after three injections, consider further imaging studies.

Achilles Bursa/Retrocalcaneal Bursa

Name of Procedure

The name of this procedure is Achilles/retrocalcaneal bursa injection.

CPT

The Current Procedural Terminology code is 20605 (injection of intermediate joint or bursa).

Indications

Achilles bursitis or retrocalcaneal bursitis is the indication for this injection. This can be a first-line treatment for Achilles/retrocalcaneal bursitis, or it can be a treatment offered after a patient has had a course of NSAIDs, changing to low-heeled shoes, and/or physical therapy.

Symptoms

- Pain over the posterior heel.
- Pain with walking up stairs or up hills.
- Symptoms worse with repetitive plantarflexion (especially running or walking up steps).

Physical Examination Findings

- Pain with direct palpation over the Achilles bursa.
- Swelling may be present around the bursa.
- Pain with active plantarflexion or passive dorsiflexion of the foot.
- Pain standing on toes.

Medications to Inject

A corticosteroid and local anesthetic mixture is injected.

Amount to Inject

The injectate amount is 2–4 mL.

Size and Gauge of Needle

A 1½-inch 25-gauge needle is used.

Local Anatomy

The Achilles bursa lies beneath the Achilles tendon (insertion of the gastrocsoleus group of muscles to the posterior calcaneus) between the Achilles tendon and the posterior tibia or posterior calcaneus. The bursa may be singular or multisegmented (a series of sacs).

Patient Position

The patient lies in the prone position with the affected foot hanging off the end of the examination table and slightly dorsiflexed.

How and Where to Inject

Direct the needle to the point of maximal tenderness of the Achilles bursa (Figures 5–13 and 5–14). The needle is inserted medial or lateral to the tendon at a right angle to the

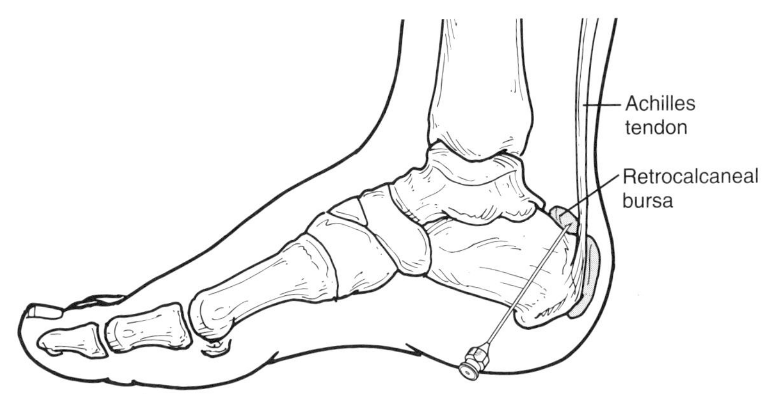

Fig 5–13 Retrocalcaneal bursa injection

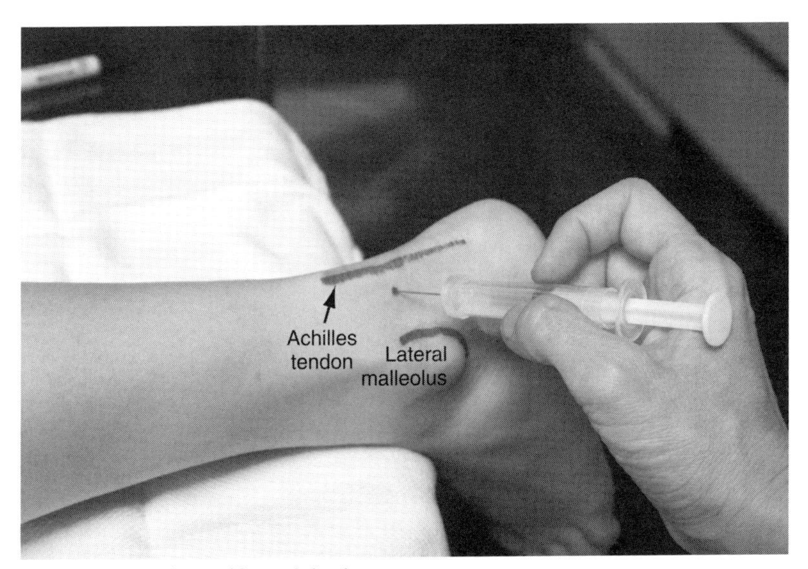

Fig 5–14 Retrocalcaneal bursa injection.

Achilles tendon, so as to avoid the tendon. The needle is directed toward the posterior tibia or calcaneus (depending on the location of maximal tenderness). The needle must remain anterior to the Achilles tendon. Inject directly into the bursa, which lies in close proximity to the bone. Many clinicians find it helpful to locate the bursa by going all the way to the bone and then pulling back approximately ¼ inch. If the needle hits the bone, the needle is withdrawn slightly into the bursa. There should be little resistance to injection if the needle is in the bursa. If there is resistance, the needle may be in the tendon, and the position should be changed. Aspirate before injecting to ensure that infection is not present and to avoid intravascular administration.

Pitfalls/Complications

It is anticipated that the patient may have an increase in pain for a few days caused by the use of corticosteroids. Informing patients of this helps to alleviate their postinjection pain concerns. If there is no relief from the injection, consider other sources of pain (Achilles tendinitis, internal derangement of the ankle, arthritis, fracture, infection, tumor, rupture of the Achilles tendon). Also, consider whether the medication actually reached the Achilles bursa. The risk of infection can be minimized with sterile preparation of the area and aseptic technique.

Postinjection Care

Apply a sterile dressing and pressure over the injection site. Have the patient ice the affected area for 20 minutes two to three times daily for the first 24–48 hours. Then begin local heat and gentle stretching exercises several days after the injection. Avoid vigorous exercise or running for several days.

When to Perform Follow-Up Injections

Although there are no strict guidelines, a reasonable approach is to reinject in 4–6 weeks if symptoms persist or return. Partial relief of symptoms is an indication for a repeat injection. A total of three injections in a given 12-month period is the accepted standard. If significant pain relief is not obtained after three injections, consider further imaging studies.

Subcutaneous Achilles Bursa

Name of Procedure

The name of this procedure is subcutaneous Achilles bursa injection.

CPT

The Current Procedural Terminology code is 20605 (injection of intermediate joint or bursa).

Indications

Subcutaneous Achilles bursitis (retroachilleal bursitis) is the indication for this injection. This should be considered after a patient has had a change in footwear and a course of NSAIDs, correction of foot deformities, and/or physical therapy. The injection can be used for both diagnostic and therapeutic purposes.

Symptoms

- Pain over the posterior heel superficial to the Achilles tendon.
- Pain is generally aggravated with certain footwear that increases the pressure over this superficial bursa.
- More common in women and location generally corresponds to the heel counter.

Physical Examination Findings

- A swollen palpable nodule may be present (pump bump) where the heel counter meets the skin.
- Pain with direct palpation over this nodule.

Medications to Inject

A corticosteroid and local anesthetic mixture is injected.

Amount to Inject

The injectate amount is 1–2 mL.

Size and Gauge of Needle

A ⅝-inch 25-gauge needle is used.

Local Anatomy

The subcutaneous Achilles bursa (also called the retroachilleal bursa) lies between the Achilles tendon and the skin of the posterior ankle. The bursa can be irritated by local pressure and friction, as in a shoe with a heel counter that is tight fitting.

Patient Position

The patient lies in the prone position with the affected foot hanging off the end of the examination table.

How and Where to Inject

Direct the needle to the point of maximal tenderness superficial to the Achilles tendon (Figures 5–15 and 5–16). Inject directly into the bursa. There should be little resistance to injection if the needle is in the bursa. If there is resistance, the needle may be in the tendon, and the position should be changed. Aspirate before injecting to avoid intravascular administration. Because this is a superficial injection, the patient should be warned of possible skin discoloration from the corticosteroid.

Pitfalls/Complications

It is anticipated that the patient may have an increase in pain for a few days caused by the use of corticosteroids. Informing patients of this helps to alleviate their postinjection pain concerns. If there is no relief from the injection, consider other sources of pain (Achilles tendinitis, internal derangement of the ankle, arthritis, calcaneal stress fracture, tarsal tunnel syndrome, infection, tumor, rheumatoid arthritis). Also, consider whether the medication actually reached the bursa. The risk of infection can be minimized with sterile preparation of the area and aseptic technique.

Postinjection Care

Apply a sterile dressing and pressure over the injection site. Have the patient ice the affected area for 20 minutes two to three times daily for the first 24–48 hours. Then begin local heat and gentle stretching exercises several days after the injection. Avoid vigorous

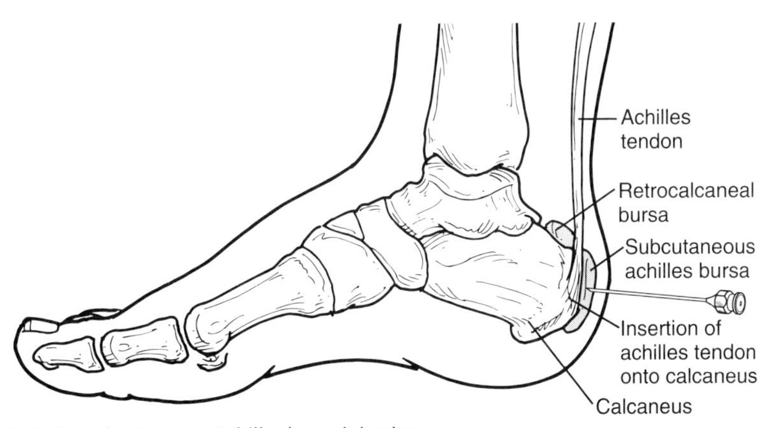

Fig 5–15 Subcutaneous Achilles bursa injection.

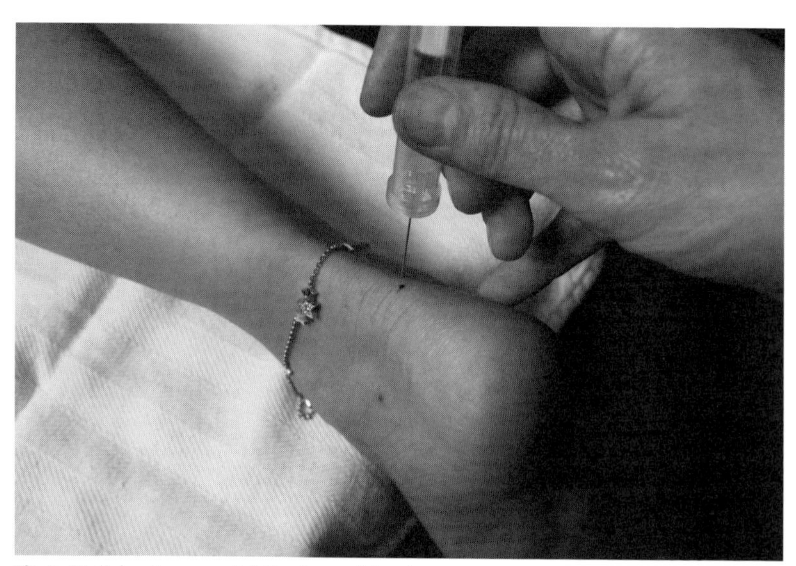

Fig 5–16 Subcutaneous Achilles bursa injection.

exercise or running for several days. Encourage the patient to discontinue the use of any footwear that may be aggravating the condition.

When to Perform Follow-Up Injections

Although there are no strict guidelines, a reasonable approach is to reinject in 4–6 weeks if symptoms persist or return. Partial relief of symptoms is an indication for a repeat injection. A total of three injections in a given 12-month period is the accepted standard. If significant pain relief is not obtained after three injections, consider further imaging studies.

6

Nerves

The injection procedures here are based on a review of the various techniques described in the medical literature as well as the authors' experiences. The techniques chosen are felt to be the most appropriate in most cases. As clinical circumstances may differ, other approaches may be more appropriate for individual cases. The reader is encouraged to familiarize himself/herself with the additional sources in the bibliography at the end of this chapter for additional approaches.

All procedures should be performed using appropriate preparation and aseptic technique. Local anesthesia (either injected or vapo-coolant spray) may be helpful in most procedures. As always, the clinician should weigh the risks and benefits of any interventional procedure.

Suprascapular Nerve

Name of Procedure

The name of this procedure is suprascapular nerve block.

CPT

The Current Procedural Terminology code is unilateral 64450 (anesthetic agent—peripheral nerve) and neurolytic 64640 (pheno neurolysis—peripheral nerve).

Indications

Nerve blocks of the suprascapular nerve can be a first-line treatment for suprascapular neuropathies, cancer pain, postoperative shoulder pain, or to facilitate shoulder range of motion in patients with adhesive capsulitis. Wearing heavy backpacks or direct injury to the nerve (frequently seen in football or trampoline injuries) can cause suprascapular nerve entrapment. It can be used as a diagnostic tool (if an anesthetizing agent is being used). Neurolytic blocks of the suprascapular nerve can be used to treat spasticity of the infraspinatus and supraspinatus muscles. Noninvasive treatments for spasticity such as medication, stretching, serial casting, icing, electrical stimulation, and positioning should be attempted before the use of neurolytic blocks. It is advisable to use a trial of botulinum toxin to the muscle before attempting neurolysis. In this way, the patient can assess the effects of a reversible procedure before an irreversible procedure is performed.

Symptoms

- Pain, usually described as deep and aching that radiates from the scapula to the shoulder.
- May have weakness or decreased range of motion of the shoulder.
- May have pain on shoulder movement, especially reaching across the chest.
- Spasticity of the supraspinatus muscle.

Physical Examination Findings

- Tenderness over the suprascapular notch.
- Spasticity of the supraspinatus muscle.
- Decreased range of motion or weakness of the shoulder may be present.
- Atrophy of the supraspinatus and infraspinatus muscle may be present.

Medications to Inject

A local anesthetic with corticosteroid or neurolytic solution is injected.

Amount to Inject

The injectate amount is 8–10 mL.

Size and Gauge of Needle

A 1½-inch 25-gauge needle is used.

Local Anatomy

The suprascapular nerve enters into the supraspinous fossa below the transverse scapular ligament. The nerve can become compressed as it passes through the suprascapular notch. The suprascapular artery and vein pass through the suprascapular notch with the nerve. The nerve innervates the supraspinatus and infraspinatus muscles. The suprascapular nerve originates from C5 and C6 spinal roots. It is a branch of the superior trunk of the brachial plexus.

Patient Position

The patient is seated with his/her back to the examiner and touching the opposite shoulder with the affected arm.

How and Where to Inject

Insert the needle ½-inch superior to a point along the scapular spine approximately 2 inches from the lateral border of the acromion (Figures 6–1 and 6–2). Insert the needle until the bone is contacted, and then withdraw slightly. Walk the needle tip along the scapula until the suprascapular notch is identified. Inject slightly cephalad into the supraspinatus fossa. The goal is to have the needle in the epineural space. Do not inject into the nerve—withdraw the needle slightly. Always aspirate before injecting to ensure that you are not in a blood vessel. Do not inject forcefully because it is a fixed space and nerve trauma may result. Inject slowly.

Pitfalls/Complications

Because of the proximity of the pleural cavity, pneumothorax is a potential complication (incidence of <1%). The patient may experience persistent paresthesia secondary to needle trauma to the nerve. Intravascular injection (specifically the suprascapular artery and vein) can be avoided by aspirating before injecting. If there is no relief from the injection, consider other sources of pain (bursitis, tendinitis, shoulder arthritis, C5 radiculopathy, Parsonage–Turner syndrome, tumor, infection). The risk of infection can be minimized with sterile preparation of the area and aseptic technique.

Postinjection Care

Apply pressure over the injection site. Have the patient ice the affected area for 20 minutes two to three times daily for the first 24–48 hours. Then begin local heat and gentle stretching exercises several days after the injection. Because the shoulder joint may be insensate

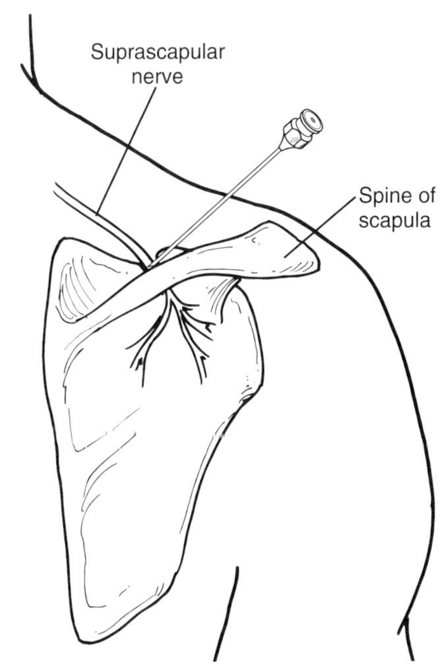

Fig 6–1 Suprascapular nerve injection.

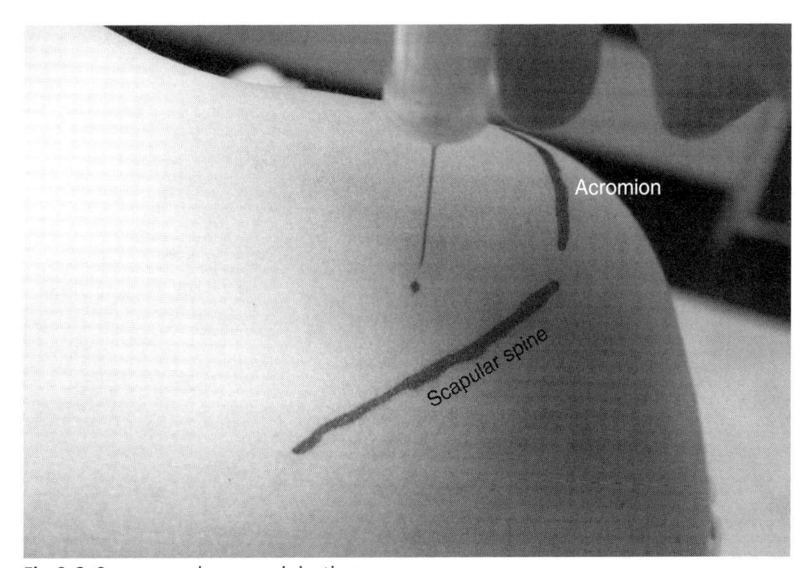

Fig 6–2 Suprascapular nerve injection.

after injection, avoid deep heat modalities and only perform supervised range of motion exercises. Avoid vigorous exercise or overhead activities for several days.

When to Perform Follow-Up Injections

Although there are no strict guidelines, a reasonable approach is to reinject in 4–6 weeks if symptoms persist or return. Partial relief of symptoms is an indication for a repeat injection. Do not inject more than once per visit because warning paresthesias may not present immediately. A total of three injections in a given 12-month period is the accepted standard.

Musculocutaneous Nerve

Name of Procedure

The name of this procedure is musculocutaneous nerve block.

CPT

The Current Procedural Terminology code is unilateral 64450 (anesthetic agent—peripheral nerve) and neurolytic 64640 (pheno neurolysis—peripheral nerve).

Indications

Because the musculocutaneous nerve innervates the biceps, coracobrachialis, and brachialis muscles, a nerve block can be used to treat spasticity in these muscles. Noninvasive treatments for spasticity such as medication, stretching, serial casting, icing, electrical stimulation, and positioning should be attempted before the use of neurolytic blocks. It is advisable to assess the effects of botulinum toxin injections in the affected muscle before attempting neurolysis. In this way, the patient can assess the effects of a reversible procedure before an irreversible procedure is performed.

Symptoms

- Difficulty in dressing secondary to spasticity (the arm may be adducted with elbow flexion).

Physical Examination Findings

- Spasticity of the biceps, brachialis, and/or coracobrachialis muscle.

Medications to Inject

A local anesthetic or neurolytic solution is injected.

Amount to Inject

The injectate amount is 3–5 mL.

Size and Gauge of Needle

A 1½-inch 23-guage needle is used.

Local Anatomy

The musculocutaneous nerve is composed of fibers from C5, C6, and C7. The nerve is derived from the upper and middle trunks, anterior division, and lateral cord of the brachial plexus. The nerve pierces the coracobrachialis muscle and then continues between the biceps and brachialis muscles in the arm. It supplies the coracobrachialis, biceps, and brachialis muscles. The musculocutaneous nerve terminates as a cutaneous branch (lateral cutaneous nerve of the forearm), which supplies the radial surface of the forearm.

Patient Position

The patient is seated comfortably, facing the examiner.

How and Where to Inject

Insert the needle below the tendon of the pectoralis major muscle (Figures 6–3 and 6–4). This is anterior to the axillary artery, which should be palpated to avoid injecting into the artery. Advance the needle toward the coracoid process, parallel to the arm. Use a nerve stimulator to confirm that the musculocutaneous nerve (and not the median nerve, which is in close proximity) is being stimulated. Confirmation that the musculocutaneous nerve is being stimulated will be noted if the patient contracts the biceps muscle. (If the median nerve is being stimulated, the patient will contract the wrist and finger flexors.) The goal is to have the needle in the muscle at the point where the nerve enters the muscle and to have the needle in the epineural space. If the needle contacts the nerve, the patient may feel paresthesia in the distribution of the nerve. Do not inject into the nerve—withdraw the needle slightly. Avoid the axillary artery by palpating this artery. Always aspirate before injecting to ensure that you are not in a blood vessel. Do not inject forcefully because it is a fixed space and nerve trauma may result. Inject slowly. The lateral cutaneous nerve of the forearm can be blocked at the elbow by injecting

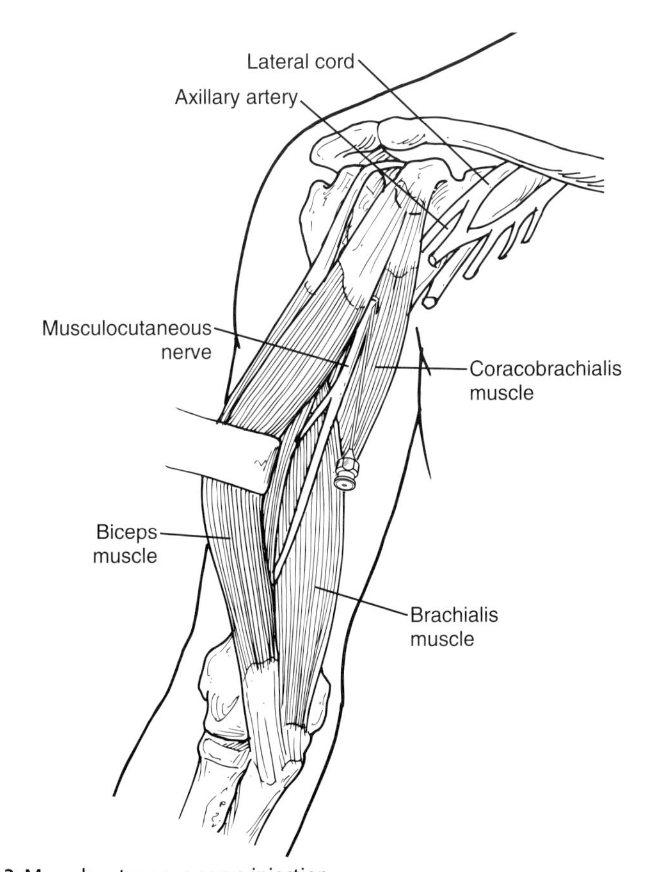

Fig 6–3 Musculocutaneous nerve injection.

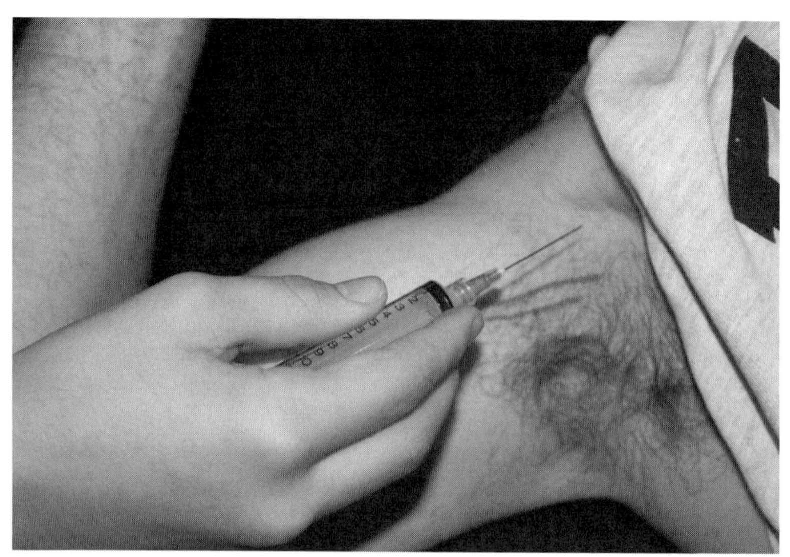

Fig 6–4 Musculocutaneous nerve injection.

lateral to the biceps tendon at the elbow crease. The injected material is delivered diffusely throughout the area.

Pitfalls/Complications

The patient may experience persistent paresthesia secondary to needle trauma to the nerve. Intravascular injection can be avoided by palpating the location of the axillary artery and aspirating before injecting. If there is no relief from the injection, consider other sources of spasticity (generalized spasticity is usually more effectively treated with systemic medications). The risk of infection can be minimized with sterile preparation of the area and aseptic technique.

Postinjection Care

Apply pressure over the injection site. Have the patient ice the affected area for 20 minutes two to three times daily for the first 24–48 hours. A therapy program for arm stretching should be initiated.

When to Perform Follow-Up Injections

Although there are no strict guidelines, a reasonable approach is to reinject in 4–6 weeks if symptoms persist or return. Partial relief of symptoms is an indication for a repeat injection. Do not inject more than once per visit, since warning paresthesias may not present immediately. A total of three injections in a given 12-month period is the accepted standard.

Greater and Lesser Occipital Nerve

Name of Procedure

The name of this procedure is greater or lesser occipital nerve block.

CPT

The Current Procedural Terminology code is unilateral 64450 (anesthetic agent—peripheral nerve).

Indications

A greater occipital nerve block can be used as a therapeutic tool to treat posterior occipital headaches caused by pressure on the greater and/or lesser occipital nerve (occipital neuralgia). Whiplash injuries may predispose to pain in the occipital region. It can be used as a diagnostic tool (if an anesthetizing agent is being used) to differentiate occipital neuralgia from cervicogenic headaches. The site of compression in occipital neuralgia can be anywhere along the nerve's course.

Symptoms

- Headaches in the region of the greater occipital nerve distribution (posterior skull), usually unilaterally.
- Pain may be referred into the facial areas.
- Headaches may be acute or chronic and may present as sudden, shocklike paresthesias.
- Patient may have a history of cervical or occipital trauma.
- Nausea, vomiting, and photophobia may be associated with the headaches.

Physical Examination Findings

- Pain on palpation of the occipital nerve.
- Local muscle spasm or trigger points may by present.
- Cervical range of motion may be limited.
- Spurling's maneuver may be positive if the source of compression of the nerve is at the C2 level.
- Palpation of the nerve on the superior nuchal line with neck flexion may exacerbate the symptoms if the source of compression of the nerve is at the tendinous insertion of the trapezius muscle.

Medications to Inject

A local anesthetic with corticosteroid is injected.

Amount to Inject

The injectate amount is 5 mL.

Size and Gauge of Needle

A 1–1½-inch 25-guage needle is used.

Local Anatomy

The greater occipital nerve is a branch of the C2 dorsal ramus and is the largest purely afferent nerve in the body. The nerve crosses deep to the semispinalis capitis muscle and emerges in the back of the head above the superior nuchal line. It enters the scalp between the semispinalis capitis and trapezius muscles. The posterior occipital artery lies lateral to the nerve. The greater occipital nerve supplies sensation to the skin in the posterior skull, including the occiput and temporal areas, and to the vertex and ear.

The lesser occipital nerve is derived from the anterior divisions of C2 and C3. It ascends along the sternocleidomastoid muscle and provides sensation to the scalp lateral to the greater occipital nerve in the lateral occipital region and posterior aspect of the ear.

Patient Position

The patient is seated with his/her back to the examiner. The neck should be flexed with the forehead resting on a pillow.

How and Where to Inject

Identify the occipital protuberance and mastoid process (Figures 6–5 and 6–6). The greater occipital nerve should lie on the medial third between these two areas, along the superior nuchal line and medial to the occipital artery. The lesser occipital nerve lies at the junction of the middle and outer third of a line between the occipital protuberance and the mastoid process. Inject into the subcutaneous tissue over the occipital bone. Inject diffusely, trying to distribute the medication in as large an area as possible. If the needle contacts the nerve, the patient may feel paresthesia in the distribution of the nerve. Do not

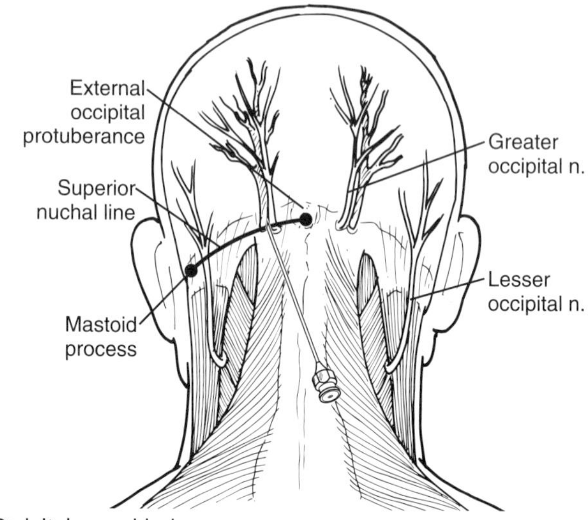

Fig 6–5 Occipital nerve block.

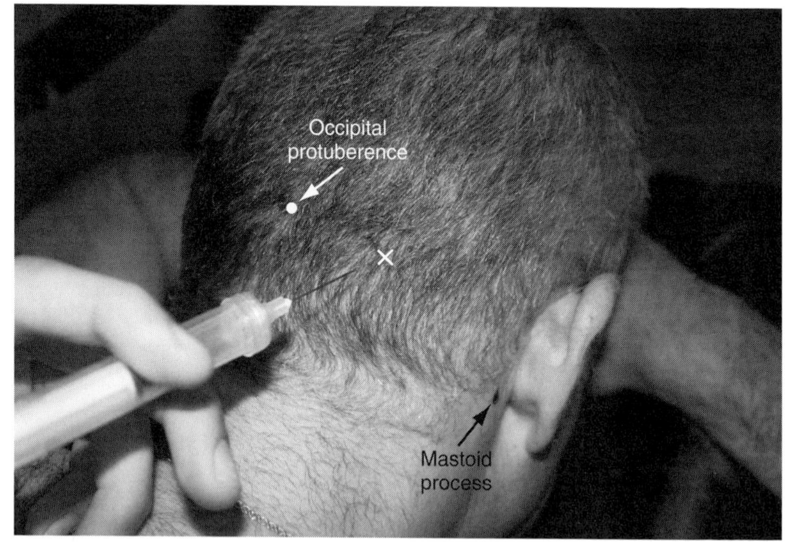

Fig 6–6 Occipital nerve block.

inject into the nerve—withdraw the needle slightly. Always aspirate before injecting to ensure that you are not in the posterior occipital artery because this runs adjacent to the nerve. Do not inject forcefully because it is a fixed space and nerve trauma may result. Inject slowly.

Pitfalls/Complications

The patient may experience persistent paresthesia secondary to needle trauma to the nerve. Intravascular injection can be avoided by aspirating before injecting. If there is no relief from the injection, consider other sources of pain (C2 radiculopathy, headaches of other origin [especially tension headaches], tumor, rheumatoid arthritis, cervical myelopathy). The risk of infection can be minimized with sterile preparation of the area and aseptic technique.

Postinjection Care

Apply pressure over the injection site. Have the patient ice the affected area for 20 minutes two to three times daily for the first 24–48 hours.

When to Perform Follow-Up Injections

Although there are no strict guidelines, a reasonable approach is to reinject in 4–6 weeks if symptoms persist or return. Partial relief of symptoms is an indication for a repeat injection. Do not inject more than once per visit because warning paresthesias may not present immediately. A total of three injections in a given 12-month period is the accepted standard.

Medial Antebrachial Cutaneous Nerve

Name of Procedure

The name of this procedure is medial antebrachial cutaneous nerve (MACN) block.

CPT

The Current Procedural Terminology code is unilateral 64450 (anesthetic agent—peripheral nerve).

Indications

This injection can be both diagnostic and therapeutic.

Symptoms

- Paresthesias or dysesthesias in the medial forearm.
- The MACN distribution will not include the ulnar aspect of the hand, and this may help distinguish it from a C8, lower trunk, or medial cord lesion.

Physical Examination Findings

- Decreased sensation in the medial forearm.
- No evidence of motor involvement.
- Sensation in the ulnar aspect of the hand should be normal.
- The sensory examination in the MACN may be completely normal as the primary symptoms (paresthesias or dysesthesia) are subjective.

Medications to Inject

A local anesthetic with corticosteroid for a therapeutic block or lidocaine alone for diagnostic block is injected.

Amount to Inject

The injectate amount is 5–7 mL.

Size and Gauge of Needle

A ⅝-inch 25- to 27-gauge needle is used.

Local Anatomy

The fibers of the MACN are derived from the lower cervical nerve roots (C8, T1) and travel through the medial cord of the brachial plexus. This sensory nerve crosses the medial aspect of the elbow medial to the biceps tendon and supplies sensation to the medial forearm. The ulnar nerve supplies the medial (ulnar) aspect of the hand.

Patient Position

The patient lies supine or sitting with the elbow flexed approximately 45 degrees.

How and Where to Inject

The insertion of the biceps tendon and the medial epicondyle are important landmarks in this injection (Figures 6–7 and 6–8). The injection is made approximately 5–6 cm proximal to the midpoint of the biceps tendon insertion and medial epicondyle. The injection should be spread out over this area. The nerve is superficial to the brachial fascia. Aspirate before injecting to avoid intravascular administration.

Pitfalls/Complications

If the injection is given too deep (beneath the brachial fascia), the nerve will not be blocked. As always, if paresthesias are elicited, slight repositioning of the needle is necessary to avoid intraneural injection. If there is no relief from the injection, consider other sources of pain (sensory only radiculopathy).

Postinjection Care

Apply pressure and ice (optional) over the injection site. Avoid vigorous exercise for several days. The patient should be prepared for a nerve anesthesia after injection.

When to Perform Follow-Up Injections

If the injection failed to elicit anesthesia, a repeat injection should be performed as soon as possible. The length of response to a successful injection and whether the injection was diagnostic or therapeutic will dictate the need for further injections.

Lateral Antebrachial Cutaneous Nerve

Name of Procedure

The name of this procedure is lateral antebrachial cutaneous nerve block.

CPT

The Current Procedural Terminology code is unilateral 64450 (anesthetic agent—peripheral nerve).

Indications

The indication for this injection is entrapment of the lateral antebrachial cutaneous nerve (LACN). This injection can be both diagnostic and therapeutic, especially in cases of refractory lateral epicondylitis.

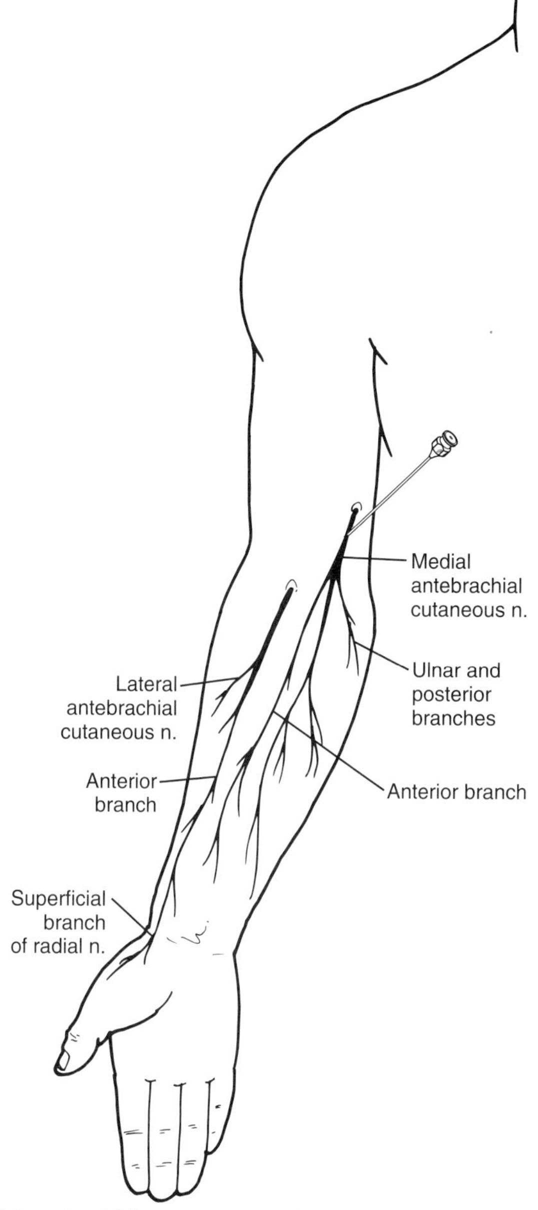

Fig 6–7 Medial antebrachial cutaneous nerve injection.

Symptoms

- Pain and/or paresthesias radiating from the elbow to the base of the thumb or a pain in the lateral aspect of the forearm.
- Lateral antebrachial cutaneous nerve (LACN) entrapment may be misdiagnosed as lateral epicondylitis and may be responsible for some cases of refractory lateral epicondylitis (tennis elbow).

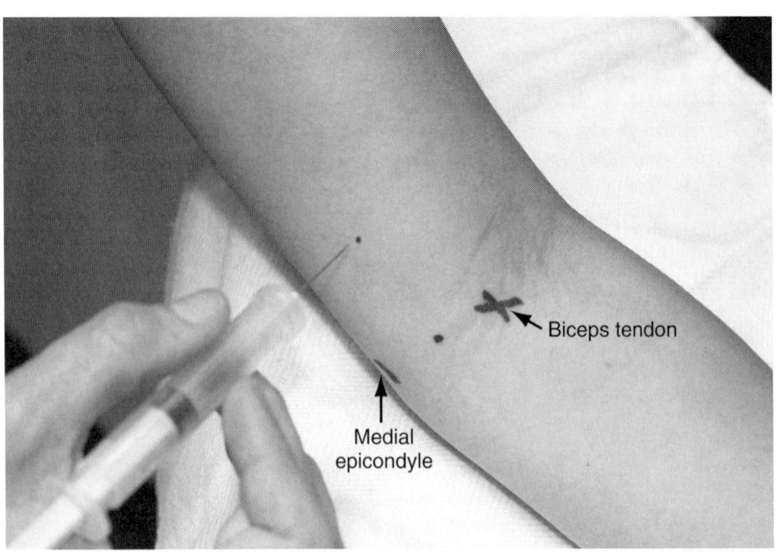

Fig 6–8 Medial antebrachial cutaneous nerve injection.

Physical Examination Findings

- In LACN entrapment, the area of greatest tenderness is not over the lateral epicondyle, but lateral to the biceps tendon at the elbow level.
- Pain may occur on resisted flexion of the forearm. It may be difficult to distinguish this from lateral epicondylitis because resisted wrist extension may also recreate pain.

Medications to Inject

A lidocaine/corticosteroid solution for therapeutic block or lidocaine alone for diagnostic block is injected.

Amount to Inject

The injectate amount is 3–7 mL.

Size and Gauge of Needle

A 1–1½-inch 25-gauge needle is used.

Local Anatomy

The LACN is a sensory nerve that is a continuation of the musculocutaneous nerve. It receives innervation from the upper cervical nerve roots (C5, C6). The fibers travel through the lateral cord of the brachial plexus. At the elbow, the nerve travels lateral to the biceps tendon. Here, the radial nerve may be in close proximity to the LACN. The LACN divides into an anterior and posterior branch. The posterior branch supplies sensation to the lateral forearm. The anterior branch supplies sensation to the base of the thumb.

Patient Position

The patient lies supine with the elbow almost fully extended.

How and Where to Inject

Just lateral to the biceps tendon, at the level of the elbow crease, insert the needle approximately one-half to three-quarters of an inch (Figures 6–9 and 6–10). If paresthesias occur, the needle is slightly repositioned, and the medication is injected. Aspirate before injecting to avoid intravascular administration.

Pitfalls/Complications

The main complications are intravascular and intraneural injections. The radial nerve may also be inadvertently blocked. If the injection is on the wrong side of the brachial

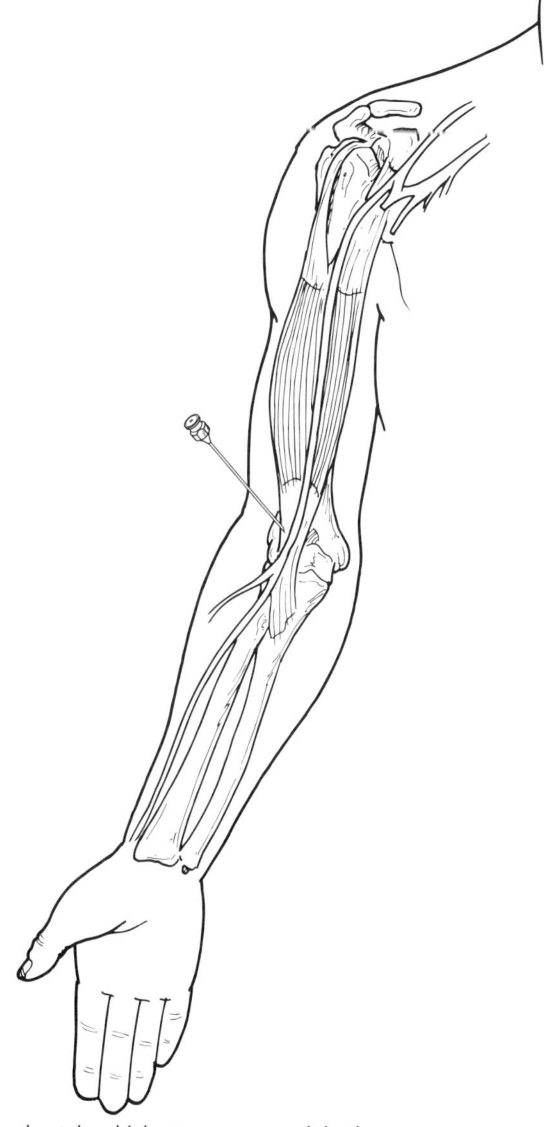

Fig 6–9 Lateral antebrachial cutaneous nerve injection.

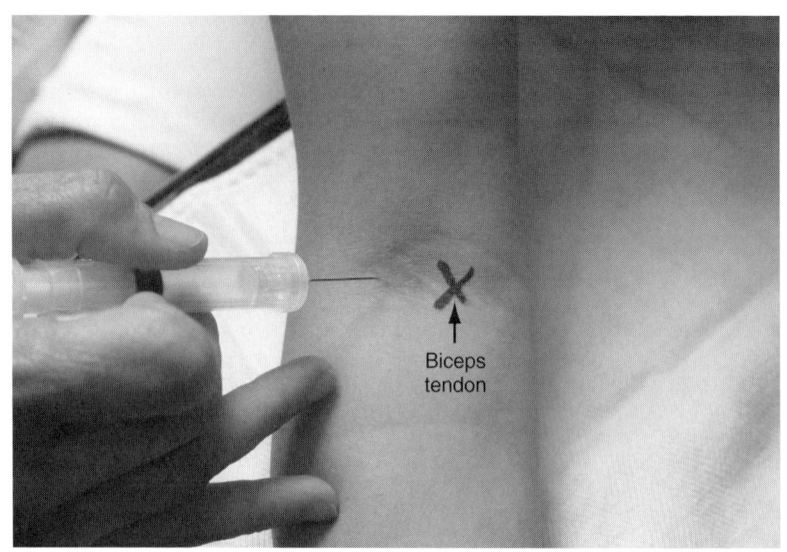

Fig 6–10 Lateral antebrachial cutaneous nerve injection.

fascia (the LACN pierces the brachial fascia around this level, but the exact location can vary), the injection is likely to fail. This will be apparent on a postinjection assessment for anesthesia. If there is no relief from the injection, consider other sources of pain (sensory only radiculopathy).

Postinjection Care

Apply pressure and ice (optional) over the injection site. Avoid vigorous exercise for several days. The patient should be prepared for a nerve anesthesia after injection.

When to Perform Follow-Up Injections

If the injection failed to elicit anesthesia, a repeat injection should be performed. The length of response to a successful injection and whether the injection was diagnostic or therapeutic will dictate the need for further injections.

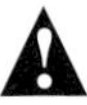

Radial Nerve Injection at the Elbow

Name of Procedure

The name of this procedure is radial nerve/posterior interosseous nerve block.

CPT

The Current Procedural Terminology code is 64550 (anesthetic agent—peripheral nerve).

Indications

Lateral epicondylitis may mimic posterior interosseous nerve entrapment at the elbow. In instances where lateral epicondylitis does not respond to conservative treatment, including injections of the lateral epicondyle, a diagnostic and therapeutic radial nerve injection at the elbow may be indicated.

Symptoms

- Pain just below the lateral epicondyle.
- Pain may commence or increase after repetitive use of the arm.
- Forearm weakness (either caused by true neurologic weakness or pain) may be present.

Physical Examination Findings

- Tenderness just below the lateral epicondyle.
- The presentation may be identical or very similar to lateral epicondylitis.

Medications to Inject

A local anesthetic for a purely diagnostic block or corticosteroid and local anesthetic for a diagnostic and therapeutic block is injected.

Amount to Inject

The injectate amount is 5–10 mL.

Size and Gauge of Needle

A 1½-inch 25-gauge needle is used.

Local Anatomy

At the level of the elbow, the radial nerve is located in the lateral antecubital fossa, between the biceps tendon and the brachioradialis muscle. In this area, the radial nerve divides into its two main branches—the posterior interosseous nerve and the superficial radial nerve. The former is primarily a motor nerve, whereas the latter is primarily sensory, although the superficial radial nerve may supply the extensor carpi radialis brevis muscle.

Patient Position

The arm is supported, and the forearm is supinated.

How and Where to Inject

The needle is inserted between the biceps tendon and the brachioradialis muscle (lateral to the biceps tendon and medial to the brachioradialis at the elbow crease) (Figures 6–11 and 6–12). The needle should be directed posteriorly toward the lateral epicondyle of the humerus. The radial nerve may be encountered at a depth of 1–1½ inches. If the bone is contacted, the needle should be slightly withdrawn, and 2–3 cc of solution should be injected. The needle should be withdrawn and reinserted in slightly different tracks medially and laterally to the first injection, and an additional 2–3 cc of solution should be injected in those areas. Care should be taken to assess for paresthesias. If paresthesias occur, a slight repositioning is necessary, and injection should be performed at that point. The goal is to inject near the nerve but not into the nerve. If there is resistance to injection, the needle may be too far medial and in the biceps tendon. Aspiration should be performed to minimize the chance of an intravascular injection. Anesthesia in the radial nerve distribution will confirm the nerve block.

Pitfalls/Complications

Intravascular injection, infection, and hematoma are always possible with any injection procedure. Aseptic technique, aspirating before injecting, and pressure after injection

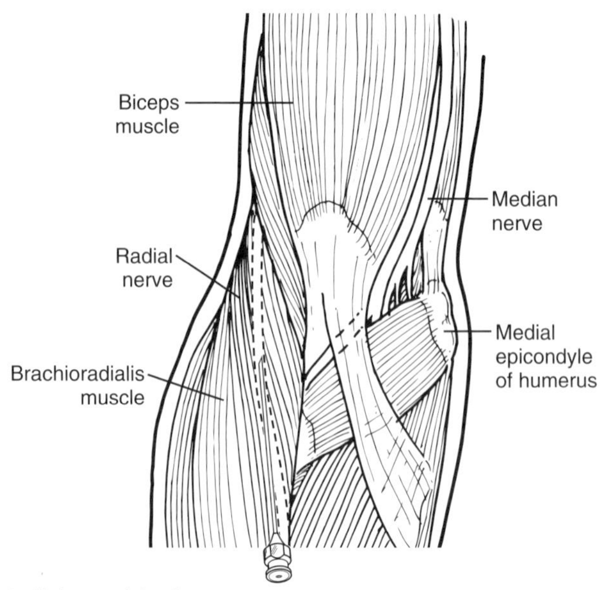

Fig 6–11 Radial nerve injection.

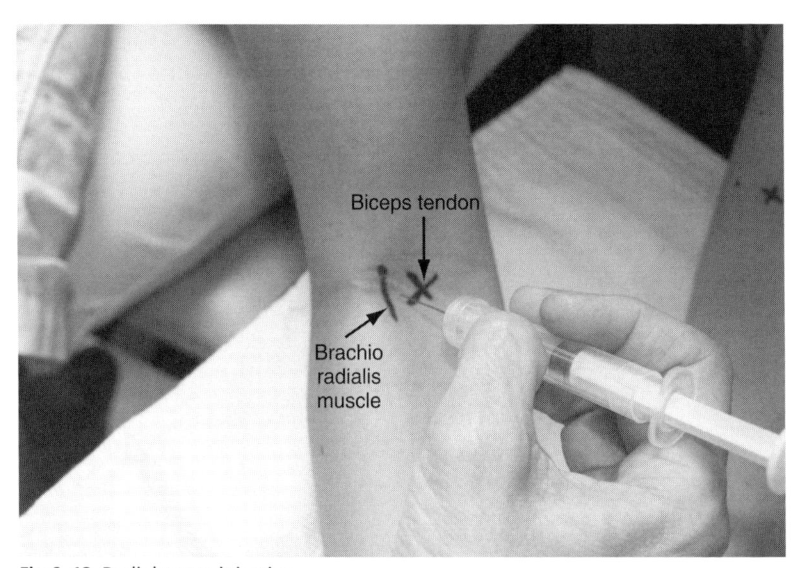

Fig 6–12 Radial nerve injection.

will help to minimize the chances of these complications. Performing the injection with a nerve stimulator may help localize the nerve and decrease the volume of fluid needed for injection. If successive effective injections are not helpful, an alternate diagnosis should be considered (lateral epicondylitis, cervical radiculopathy, radial tunnel syndrome, arthritis, fracture, triceps tendinitis, bursitis, elbow synovitis).

Postinjection Care

Apply pressure over the area of the injection. Use ice to minimize pain and swelling. Avoid heavy exercise with the forearm for several days.

When to Perform Follow-Up Injections

If anesthesia was not obtained in a radial distribution, it is likely the injection missed its mark. A repeat injection should be performed. Electrical stimulation for localization should probably be considered for any subsequent injection. If the initial injection used only local anesthetic (assuming anesthesia and posterior interosseous nerve weakness was obtained) and symptoms persist, an additional injection with corticosteroid would be indicated. A total of three injections in a given 12-month period is the accepted standard.

Median Nerve Injection at the Wrist (Carpal Tunnel Injection)

Name of Procedure

The name of this procedure is median nerve block.

CPT

The Current Procedural Terminology code is unilateral 64450 (anesthetic agent—peripheral nerve).

Indications

The indication for this injection is carpal tunnel syndrome (CTS). This injection can be both diagnostic and therapeutic. An injection is usually indicated after a course of splinting and/or nonsteroidal anti-inflammatories has failed and before surgery is considered.

Symptoms

- Hand pain and numbness, especially at night.
- Symptoms may wake the patient from sleep.
- Symptoms may be in a median distribution (digits 1–3 and radial half of digit 4), but most patients report symptoms in the entire hand.
- Symptoms are frequently worse with repetitive activities and with prolonged positioning (especially driving).
- Symptoms may be improved with wrist splints.
- Weakness is a less common complaint than pain and numbness but may be present.
- The patient may complain of dropping things or difficulty with activities requiring thumb movements.

Physical Examination Findings

- Sensation may be subjectively altered in a median distribution.
- Thumb abduction weakness or APB atrophy may be present (generally in advanced cases).
- Phalen's sign or reverse Phalen's sign (extreme wrist flexion or extension) may re-create symptoms. This is considered positive if it re-creates paresthesia and not merely wrist pain.
- Tinel's sign (tapping median nerve at wrist) may reproduce symptoms.
- Very often in CTS, the examination is normal, and the history is the most important factor.

Medications

A local anesthetic–corticosteroid mixture is injected. Do not use anesthetic with epinephrine.

Amount to Inject

The injectate amount is 1–3 mL.

Size and Gauge of Needle

A 1½-inch 25-gauge needle is used.

Local Anatomy

(In the hand, the terms medial and lateral should not be used for localization. The terms radial and ulnar should be used to avoid confusion and ambiguity.) The tendons of the wrist are important anatomical landmarks to properly position the needle in relation to the median nerve. The wrist flexor tendons can be appreciated by resisted finger flexion and wrist flexion. The most radial prominent tendon is the flexor carpi radialis (FCR). The palmaris longus (PL) is ulnar to the FCR (the PL can be absent in up to 20% of the population). The median nerve is deep to and between the tendons of the PL and FCR.

Patient Position

The forearm is fully supinated and supported. Identify the tendons noted in the preceding.

How and Where to Inject

The needle should be inserted <1 cm proximal to the distal wrist crease between the tendons of the PL and FCR (Figures 6–13 and 6–14). If there is no PL present, the needle should be inserted slightly ulnar to the FCR tendon. It should be directed toward the middle finger at a 30- to 45-degree angle. Insert the needle approximately 1 cm. If the needle contacts bone, it should be withdrawn and directed slightly more superiorly. The patient should be prepared to report paresthesia, indicating contact with the nerve. Aspirate before injecting to avoid intravascular injection. Because the carpal tunnel (CT) is a confined space, avoid injecting if resistance is encountered. This will also help avoid intratendon or intraneural injection. The goal is to inject near the nerve but not into the nerve. If paresthesias are elicited, withdraw the needle slightly.

Pitfalls/Complications

The patient may experience paresthesia if the needle touches the nerve. The quantity of fluid can transiently increase pressure in the carpal tunnel and, therefore, temporarily increase the patient's symptoms. If no relief from injection occurs, consider an alternate diagnosis (wrist arthritis, cervical radiculopathy, brachial plexopathy, median nerve injury more proximally) or a missed injection (medication not in carpal tunnel). In very advanced CTS, there may already be severe nerve damage, and the injection may be ineffective.

Postinjection Care

Apply pressure and ice over the injection site. Avoid vigorous hand and wrist movements or exercise for several days. A night splint may be useful to avoid sleeping with the wrists held in flexion. The patient should be prepared for a median nerve anesthesia after injection.

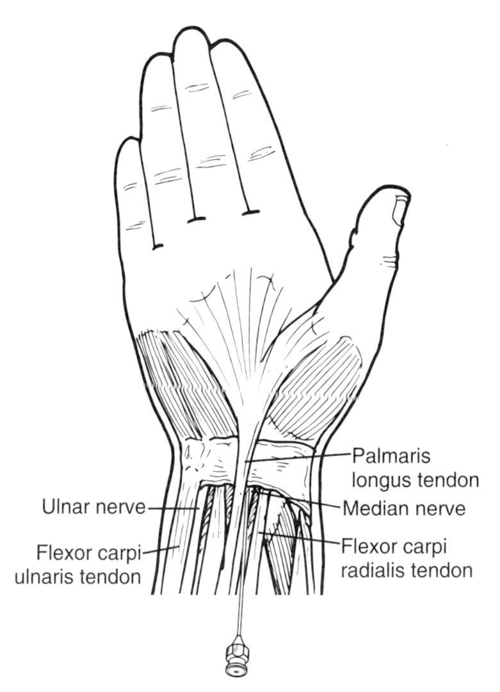

Fig 6–13 Median nerve injection in the wrist.

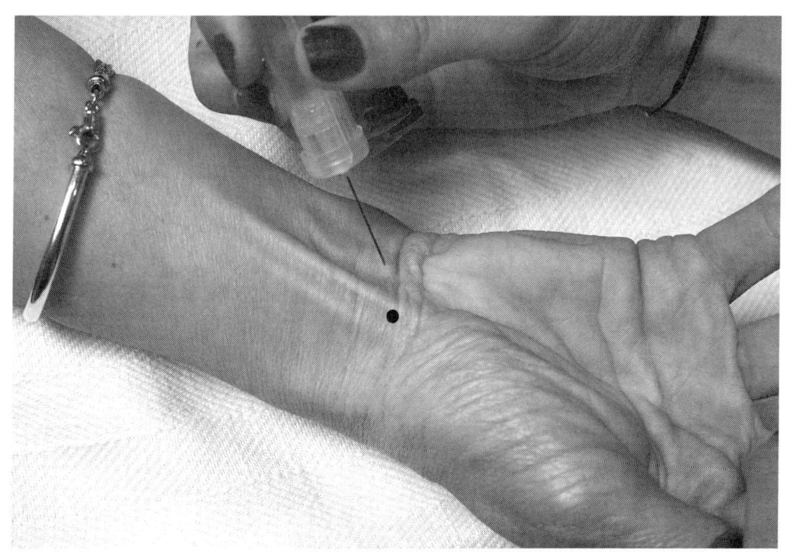

Fig 6–14 Median nerve injection in the wrist.

When to Perform Follow-Up Injections

If weeks of relief are obtained, this suggests a good response to CT release surgery. If relief lasts for months, an additional injection may be beneficial.

Ulnar Nerve at Guyon's Canal

Name of Procedure

The name of this procedure is ulnar nerve block.

CPT

The Current Procedural Terminology code is unilateral 64450 (anesthetic agent—peripheral nerve).

Indications

Injections of the ulnar nerve at Guyon's canal are usually performed after conservative management has failed. This includes rest, NSAID medication, ergonomic adjustments, therapy, and/or wrist splints.

Symptoms

- Numbness in the fourth and fifth digits.
- Pain in the wrist that radiates into the palm and dorsum of the hand on the ulnar aspect of the hand.
- Decreased strength in the hand, especially in grip strength.

Physical Examination Findings

- Sensation to the volar (palmar) aspect of the fifth digit and ulnar aspect of the fourth digit may be affected, with sparing of the dorsal aspect of these fingers. (Involvement of the dorsal aspect of the hand usually indicates a more proximal lesion.)
- Weakness of the ulnarly innervated hand muscles may be present. The strength in the flexor carpi ulnaris should be normal because the lesion is distal to the innervation of this muscle.
- Atrophy of the intrinsic muscles may be present.
- Tinel's sign may be present at the wrist (over the ulnar nerve as it passes beneath the transverse carpal ligament).

Medications to Inject

A local anesthetic with corticosteroid is injected.

Amount to Inject

The injectate amount is 1–3 mL.

Size and Gauge of Needle

A 1-inch 25-gauge needle is used.

Local Anatomy

The ulnar nerve enters the wrist below the tendon of the flexor carpi ulnaris (FCU) and proximal to the pisiform bone. Guyon's canal is composed of the pisiform bone medially and proximally and the hook of the hamate bone distally and laterally. The roof of

Guyon's canal is the deep forearm fascia. The transverse carpal ligament forms the floor of the canal. The ulnar artery and vein traverse the canal with the ulnar nerve. Within the canal, the nerve bifurcates into the deep motor branch (supplying the hypothenar muscles, the interosseous, the medial two lumbricals, the adductor pollicis, and part of the flexor pollicis brevis muscles) and the superficial branch (supplies innervation to the palmar aspect of the fifth finger and ulnar half of the fourth finger). Therefore, either the sensory and/or the motor branch may be affected in Guyon's canal entrapment. Because the dorsal ulnar cutaneous nerve branches proximal to Guyon's canal, it is not affected in ulnar nerve entrapment at the canal.

Patient Position

The hand is fully supinated.

How and Where to Inject

Have the patient flex the wrist and make a fist (Figures 6–15 and 6–16). Identify the flexor carpi ulnaris tendon. Inject on the radial side of the tendon, proximal to the wrist crease and ulnar to the ulnar artery. Angle the needle to 30 degrees, and advance the needle until it is just beyond the tendon. The patient should be prepared to report paresthesia, indicating contact with the nerve. Aspirate before injecting to avoid intravascular injection. Because Guyon's canal is a confined space, avoid injecting if resistance is encountered. This will also help avoid intratendon or intraneural injection. The goal is to

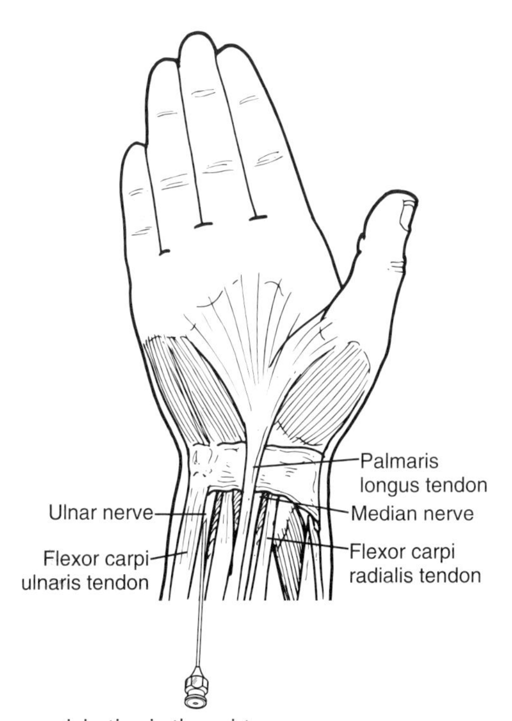

Fig 6–15 Ulnar nerve injection in the wrist.

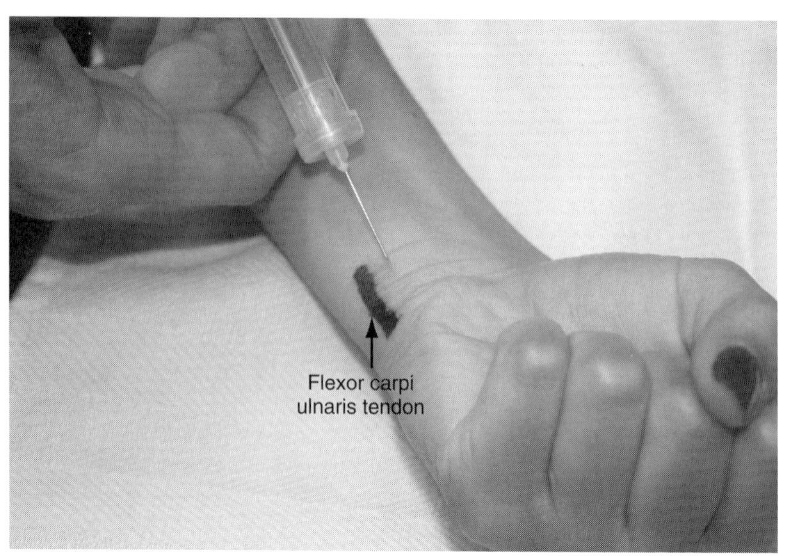

Fig 6–16 Ulnar nerve injection in the wrist.

inject near the nerve but not into the nerve. If paresthesias are elicited, withdraw the needle slightly. Do not inject forcefully because it is a fixed space and nerve trauma may result. Inject slowly.

Pitfalls/Complications

The patient may experience persistent paresthesia secondary to needle trauma to the nerve. Intravascular injection into the ulnar artery can be avoided by palpating the ulnar artery and by aspirating before injecting. If there is no relief from the injection, consider other sources of pain (ulnar nerve entrapment at a more proximal site, C8/T1 radiculopathy, lower trunk or medial cord plexopathy, carpal tunnel syndrome, peripheral neuropathy, thoracic outlet syndrome, Pancoast's tumor, peripheral neuropathy, arthritis of the carpometacarpal joints). Ganglion cysts, ulnar artery aneurysm, lipoma, or pisohamate arthritis may compress the ulnar nerve and require surgical intervention. The risk of infection can be minimized with sterile preparation of the area and aseptic technique.

Postinjection Care

Apply pressure over the injection site. Have the patient ice the affected area for 20 minutes two to three times daily for the first 24–48 hours. Then begin local heat and gentle stretching exercises several days after the injection. The hand may be splinted for several days to protect the injection site.

When to Perform Follow-Up Injections

Although there are no strict guidelines, a reasonable approach is to reinject in 4–6 weeks if symptoms persist or return. Partial relief of symptoms is an indication for a repeat injection. Do not inject more than once per visit because warning paresthesias may not present immediately. A total of three injections in a given 12-month period is the accepted standard.

Iliohypogastric Nerve Block

Name of Procedure

The name of this procedure is iliohypogastric nerve block.

CPT

The Current Procedural Terminology code is unilateral 64450 (anesthetic agent—peripheral nerve).

Indications

This injection can be both diagnostic and therapeutic. The injection may help to differentiate between iliohypogastric nerve entrapment, a high lumbar radiculopathy, or other causes of lower abdominal/groin pain.

Symptoms

- Pain, paresthesias, or numbness in the lower abdomen or groin region.

Physical Examination Findings

- The physical examination is likely to be unremarkable.
- A Tinel's sign may be present over the iliohypogastric nerve several centimeters medial to the anterior superior iliac spine (ASIS).

Medications to Inject

A lidocaine/corticosteroid solution for therapeutic block and lidocaine alone for diagnostic block are injected.

Amount to Inject

The injectate amount is 5–10 mL.

Size and Gauge of Needle

A 1½-inch 25-gauge needle is used.

Local Anatomy

The iliohypogastric nerve is derived from the L1 nerve root. The nerve travels with the ilioinguinal nerve along the abdominal wall and pierces the transverse abdominis muscle medial to the anterior superior iliac spine. The ilioinguinal nerve runs inferior to the iliohypogastric nerve. The iliohypogastric nerve innervates the skin over the lower abdominal wall toward the groin.

Patient Position

The patient lies supine.

How and Where to Inject

The injection should be made in the point approximately 3 cm medial to the anterior superior iliac spine along the line between the ASIS and the umbilicus (Figures 6–17 and 6–18). The clinician may feel a popping sensation as the needle pierces the fascia of the external oblique muscle. Anesthesia in the distribution of the iliohypogastric nerve confirms a successful nerve block. Aspirate before injecting to avoid intravascular administration.

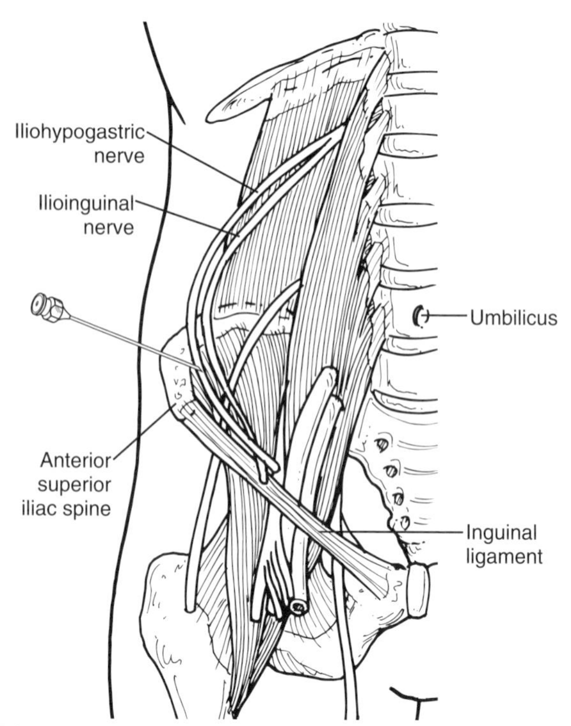

Fig 6–17 Iliohypogastric nerve injection.

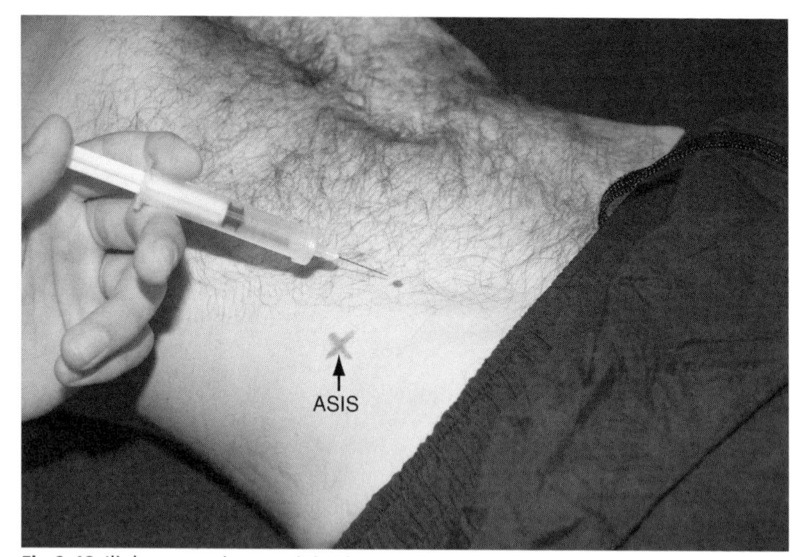

Fig 6–18 Iliohypogastric nerve injection.

Pitfalls/Complications

The peritoneal cavity and abdominal viscera lie beneath the abdominal wall. Care must be taken not to insert the needle too deep. If there is no relief from the injection, consider other sources of pain (high lumbar radiculopathy or other causes of lower abdominal/groin pain).

Postinjection Care

Apply pressure and ice (optional) over the injection site. Avoid vigorous exercise for several days. The patient should be prepared for a nerve anesthesia after injection.

When to Perform Follow-Up Injections

If the injection failed to elicit anesthesia, a repeat injection should be performed. The length of response to a successful injection and whether the injection was diagnostic or therapeutic will dictate the need for further injections.

Ilioinguinal Nerve Block

Name of Procedure

The name of this procedure is ilioinguinal nerve block.

CPT

The Current Procedural Terminology code is unilateral 64450 (anesthetic agent—peripheral nerve).

Indications

This injection can be both diagnostic and therapeutic. The injection may help to distinguish groin pain derived from ilioinguinal nerve entrapment from groin pain derived from a high lumbar radiculopathy.

Symptoms

- Pain, paresthesias, or numbness in the medial thigh, scrotum, or labium.

Physical Examination Findings

- The physical examination may be unremarkable.
- A Tinel's sign may be present over the ilioinguinal nerve several centimeters medial to the anterior superior iliac spine.

Medications to Inject

A lidocaine/corticosteroid solution is injected for a therapeutic block, and lidocaine alone is injected for a diagnostic block.

Amount to Inject

The injectate amount is 5–10 mL.

Size and Gauge of Needle

A 1½-inch 25-gauge needle is used.

Local Anatomy

The ilioinguinal nerve is derived from the L1 nerve root. The nerve travels with the iliohypogastric nerve along the abdominal wall and pierces the transverse abdominis muscle medial to the anterior superior iliac spine. The ilioinguinal nerve runs inferior to the iliohypogastric nerve. The ilioinguinal nerve enters the inguinal canal with the spermatic cord. In the male patient, it innervates the scrotum, whereas in the female patient, it innervates the labium. It also supplies sensation to the proximal medial thigh.

Patient Position

The patient lies supine.

How and Where to Inject

The injection should be made in a point approximately 3 cm medial and 3 cm inferior to the anterior superior iliac spine (Figures 6–19 and 6–20). The clinician may feel a popping sensation as the needle pierces the fascia of the external oblique muscle. Anesthesia in the distribution of the ilioinguinal nerve confirms a successful nerve block. Aspirate before injecting to avoid intravascular administration.

Pitfalls/Complications

The peritoneal cavity and abdominal viscera lie beneath the abdominal wall. Care must be taken not to insert the needle too deep. If there is no relief from the injection, consider other sources of pain (high lumbar radiculopathy, adductor muscle strain, or genital disorders).

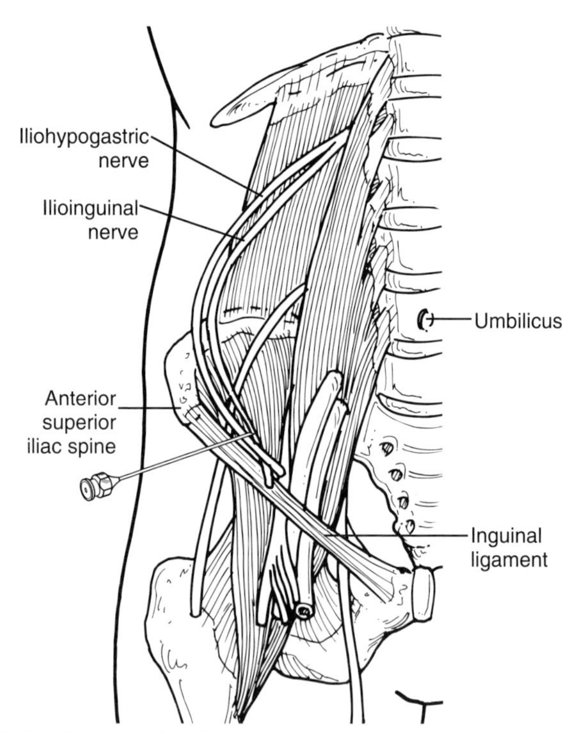

Fig 6–19 Ilioinguinal nerve injection.

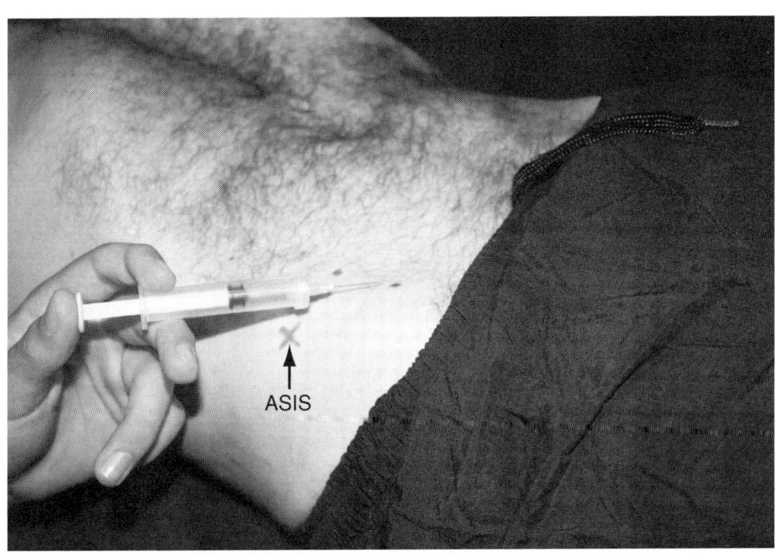

Fig 6–20 Ilioinguinal nerve injection.

Postinjection Care

Apply pressure and ice (optional) over the injection site. Avoid vigorous exercise for several days. The patient should be prepared for a nerve anesthesia after injection.

When to Perform Follow-Up Injections

If the injection failed to elicit anesthesia, a repeat injection should be performed. The length of response to a successful injection and whether the injection was diagnostic or therapeutic will dictate the need for further injections.

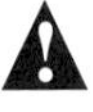

Lateral Femoral Cutaneous Nerve Injection (Meralgia Paresthetica Injection)

Name of Procedure

The name of this procedure is lateral femoral cutaneous nerve block.

CPT

The Current Procedural Terminology code is unilateral 64450 (anesthetic agent—peripheral nerve).

Indications

This injection can be both diagnostic and therapeutic. Because this is primarily a sensory nerve, neurolytic blocks are generally not used. Several electrodiagnostic techniques have been described to assess meralgia paresthetica (sensory nerve conduction studies and somatosensory evoked potentials). These studies may be technically difficult and inconclusive. For this reason, injection is likely to be a first-line treatment both from a diagnostic and therapeutic standpoint.

Symptoms

- Pain, paresthesia, or dysesthesia in the cutaneous distribution of the nerve (anterolateral or lateral thigh).
- Patient may report recent weight gain, wearing tight clothing, repetitive hip extension, or use of a tool belt around the waist.

Physical Examination Findings

- Normal motor examination.
- Hypoesthesia or dysesthesia over the anterolateral or lateral thigh.
- Tinel's sign may be elicited over the inguinal ligament approximately 2 cm medial and inferior to the ASIS.
- Paresthesias may be reproducible with hip extension.

Medications to Inject

Five to 10 mL of a local anesthetic/corticosteroid solution should be injected.

Size and Gauge of Needle

A 1½-inch 25-gauge needle with a 10-cc syringe is most commonly used. The length of the needle will depend on how much subcutaneous tissue is in the affected area. People who have more adipose tissue will require the use of a longer needle.

Local Anatomy

The lateral femoral cutaneous nerve is a purely sensory nerve and originates from the upper lumbar roots (L2, L3). The nerve runs along the lateral border of the psoas muscle, then deep to the iliac fascia on the iliacus muscle. It emerges from the muscle inferior and medial to the anterior superior iliac spine. It travels just beneath the inguinal ligament and beneath the fascia lata before dividing into a descending branch and a posterior branch. The descending branch innervates the anterolateral thigh, and the posterior branch innervates the lateral thigh. The lateral femoral cutaneous nerve provides sensation to the anterolateral aspect of the thigh. Entrapment of this nerve most commonly occurs beneath the inguinal ligament medial to the anterior superior iliac spine.

Patient Position

The patient lies supine.

How and Where to Inject

The needle is inserted approximately 1 inch medial and inferior to the anterior superior iliac spine (Figures 6–21 and 6–22). The needle insertion should be just below the inguinal ligament. It should be inserted to a depth of approximately 1 inch. Anesthesia in the lateral femoral cutaneous nerve distribution indicates a successfully placed injection. Aspirate before injecting to avoid intravascular administration.

Pitfalls/Complications

The patient may experience paresthesia if the needle touches the nerve. This can be helpful in localizing the nerve; however, intraneural injection is not desirable. Therefore, a slight withdrawal of the needle followed by injection should be performed if paresthesias in the lateral femoral cutaneous distribution are elicited. The femoral, ilioinguinal, or iliohypogastric nerves are located nearby and may be anesthetized if needle placement is incorrect or if a large volume of anesthetic is used. If there is no relief from injection,

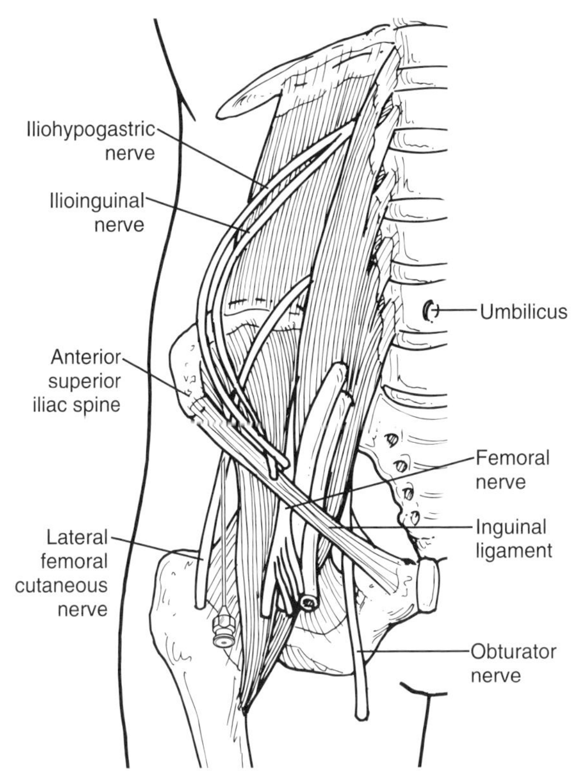

Fig 6–21 Lateral femoral cutaneous nerve injection.

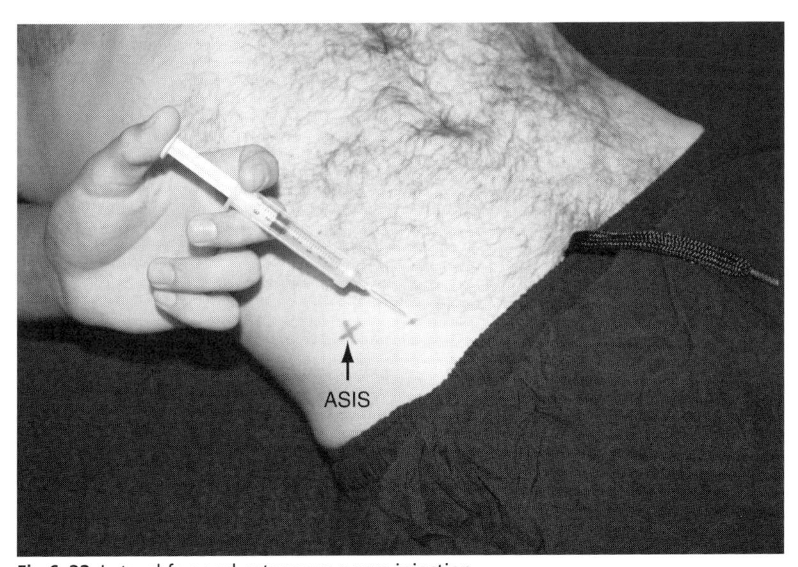

Fig 6–22 Lateral femoral cutaneous nerve injection.

consider an alternate diagnosis (upper lumbar radiculopathy, intrapelvic tumors, peripheral neuropathy, hip arthritis, trochanteric bursitis) or a missed injection.

Postinjection Care

Apply pressure and ice (optional) over the injection site. Avoid vigorous exercise for several days. The patient should be prepared for a nerve anesthesia after injection.

When to Perform Follow-Up Injections

If anesthesia was not elicited after the injection, a repeat injection in several weeks would be warranted. The limitations on repeating this type of injection are primarily related to the quantity of corticosteroid given systemically.

Obturator Nerve

Name of Procedure

The name of this procedure is obturator nerve block.

CPT

The Current Procedural Terminology code is unilateral 64450 (anesthetic agent—peripheral nerve) and neurolytic 64640 (pheno neurolysis—peripheral nerve).

Indications

Obturator nerve blocks can be used as a treatment for obturator nerve entrapment, for spasticity of the adductor muscles (neurolysis), or as a diagnostic tool (if using an anesthetizing agent). Noninvasive treatments for spasticity such as medication, stretching, serial casting, icing, electrical stimulation, and positioning should be attempted before the use of neurolytic blocks. It is advisable to try botulinum toxin to the muscle before attempting neurolysis. In this way, the patient can assess the effects of a reversible procedure before an irreversible procedure is performed.

Symptoms

Obturator nerve entrapment:

- Paresthesias, pain, and/or numbness in the medial thigh.
- Pain worse with leg extension.
- Gait disturbance caused by hip adductor weakness.

Spasticity in muscles supplied by the obturator nerve:

- Adductor muscle spasticity.
- Scissoring gait.
- Patients may complain of difficulty with perineal care, bed positioning, urinary catheterization, or sexual intercourse caused by adductor spasticity.

Physical Examination Findings

Obturator nerve entrapment:

- Hip adductor weakness may be present.
- Gait abnormality caused by hip adductor weakness (wide-based gait with hip in abduction).
- Decreased sensation in the medial thigh.

Spasticity in muscles supplied by the obturator nerve:

- Adductor muscle spasticity.
- Hyperreflexia.
- Scissoring gait.

Medications to Inject

A local anesthetic with corticosteroid (for obturator nerve entrapment) or neurolytic solution (for spasticity of muscles supplied by the obturator nerve) is injected.

Amount to Inject

The injectate amount is 10 mL.

Size and Gauge of Needle

A 3-inch 22-gauge needle is used.

Local Anatomy

The obturator nerve can become entrapped as it passes through the obturator canal. The anterior branch of the obturator nerve innervates the adductor longus, adductor brevis, and gracilis muscles, as well as giving innervation to the hip joint. The posterior branch innervates the external obturator and adductor magnus (which is dually innervated by the obturator and sciatic nerves) muscles as well as supplying innervation to the knee joint. The obturator nerve originates from posterior divisions of L2, L3, and L4 spinal roots. The obturator artery and vein travel with the obturator nerve in the obturator canal.

Patient Position

The patient lies supine with the legs slightly abducted and externally rotated.

How and Where to Inject

Palpate the pubic tubercle and insert the needle 1–2 inches laterally and inferiorly (Figures 6–23 and 6–24). When bone is contacted (the superior pubic ramus), redirect the needle slightly laterally. Advance the needle approximately 1 inch into the obturator foramen. The goal is to have the needle in the epineural space. If the needle contacts the nerve, the patient may feel paresthesia in the distribution of the nerve. Do not inject into the nerve—withdraw the needle slightly. A nerve stimulator may be used to help localize the nerve. Always aspirate before injecting to ensure that you are not in a blood vessel. Do not inject forcefully because it is a fixed space and nerve trauma may result. Inject slowly.

Pitfalls/Complications

The patient may experience persistent paresthesia secondary to needle trauma to the nerve. Intravascular injection (specifically the obturator artery and vein) can be avoided by aspirating before injecting. If the injection is too deep or misdirected, the needle could enter the bladder or vagina. If there is no relief from the injection, consider other sources of pain (tumor, hematoma, lumbar plexopathy, diabetic amyotrophy, infection, hip pathology). The risk of infection can be minimized with sterile preparation of the area and aseptic technique.

Postinjection Care

Apply pressure over the injection site. Have the patient ice the affected area for 20 minutes two to three times daily for the first 24–48 hours. Then begin local heat and gentle stretching exercises several days after the injection. Avoid vigorous exercise or running for several days.

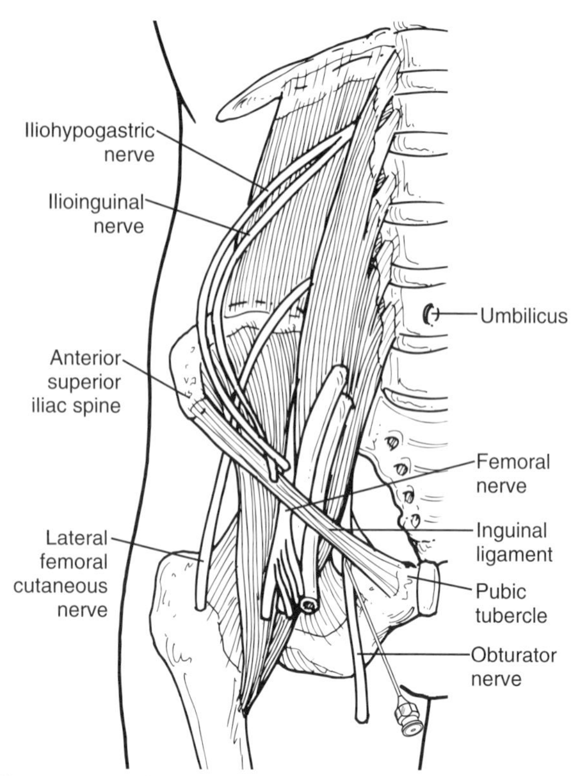

Fig 6–23 Obturator nerve injection.

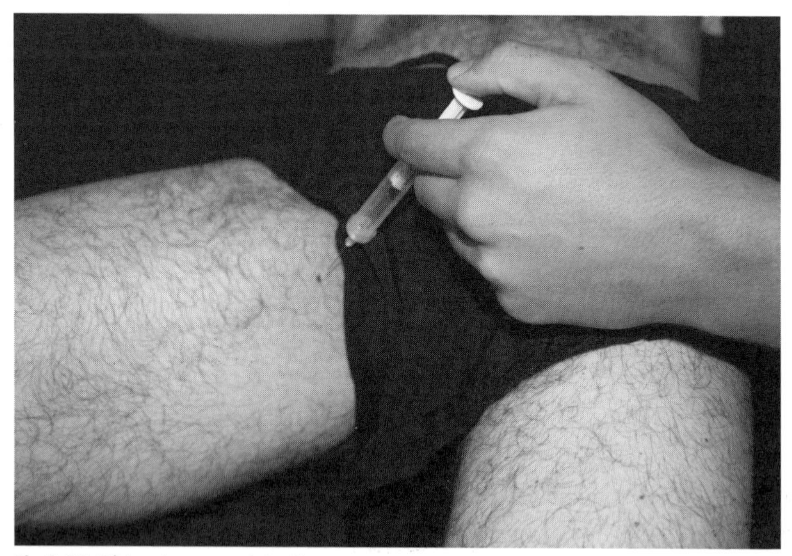

Fig 6–24 Obturator nerve injection.

When to Perform Follow-Up Injections

Although there are no strict guidelines, a reasonable approach is to reinject in 4–6 weeks if symptoms persist or return. Partial relief of symptoms is an indication for a repeat injection. Do not inject more than once per visit, since warning paresthesias may not present immediately. A total of three injections in a given 12-month period is the accepted standard.

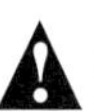

Femoral Nerve

Name of Procedure

The name of this procedure is femoral nerve block.

CPT

The Current Procedural Terminology code is unilateral 64450 (anesthetic agent—peripheral nerve) and neurolytic 64640 (pheno neurolysis—peripheral nerve).

Indications

This can be a first-line treatment for postherpetic neuralgia, postamputation pain, complex regional pain syndrome, to decrease knee pain during physical therapy, and tumor-related pain, or it can be used as a diagnostic tool (if an anesthetizing agent is used). Neurolytic blocks of the nerve can be used to treat spasticity of the quadriceps muscle. Noninvasive treatments for spasticity such as medication, stretching, serial casting, icing, electrical stimulation, and positioning should be attempted before the use of neurolytic blocks. It is advisable to use a trail of Botox to the muscle before attempting neurolysis. In this way, the patient can assess the effects of a reversible procedure before an irreversible procedure is performed.

Symptoms

- Difficulty walking secondary to severe knee extensor spasticity.
- Pain in the anterior thigh or the medial side of the leg below the knee.

Physical Examination Findings

- Severe knee extensor spasticity.
- Pain in the distribution of the femoral or saphenous nerve.

Medications to Inject

A local anesthetic with corticosteroid or neurolytic solution is injected.

Amount to Inject

The injectate amount is 10 mL.

Size and Gauge of Needle

A 1½-inch 22-guage needle is used.

Local Anatomy

The femoral nerve arises from the ventral rami of the second, third, and fourth lumbar nerves. After emerging from the psoas muscle, it passes over the iliacus muscle and then under the inguinal ligament into the thigh. Here, the nerve is immediately lateral to the femoral artery, which is lateral to the femoral vein. The nerve lies deep to the fascia lata and fascia iliacus. The nerve divides into anterior and posterior branches in the proximal anterior thigh. The anterior division supplies the cutaneous innervation to the anterior thigh and innervates the sartorius muscle. The posterior division innervates the quadriceps muscle and the knee joint and terminates as the saphenous nerve, which supplies cutaneous innervation to the medial side of the leg below the knee.

Patient Position

The patient lies supine.

How and Where to Inject

The femoral nerve is immediately lateral to the femoral artery as it travels under the inguinal ligament (Figures 6–25 and 6–26). Palpate the femoral artery just below the inguinal ligament and inject slightly laterally 1–2 cm below the inguinal ligament. There is usually a loss of resistance once the fascia lata and fascia iliaca have been pierced. Position the needle approximately 45 degrees cephalad. Some physicians prefer to use a nerve stimulator to ensure that needle placement is correct. The needle is advanced while a stimulating current of 1.0 mA, 2 Hz, and 0.1 ms is used. The needle is advanced slowly until quadriceps muscle contraction is noted. Then proceed with the injection, injecting in 5-mL increments and always aspirating before injecting so as to avoid intravascular administration.

The goal is to have the needle in the epineural space. If the needle contacts the nerve, the patient may feel paresthesia in the distribution of the nerve. Do not inject into the

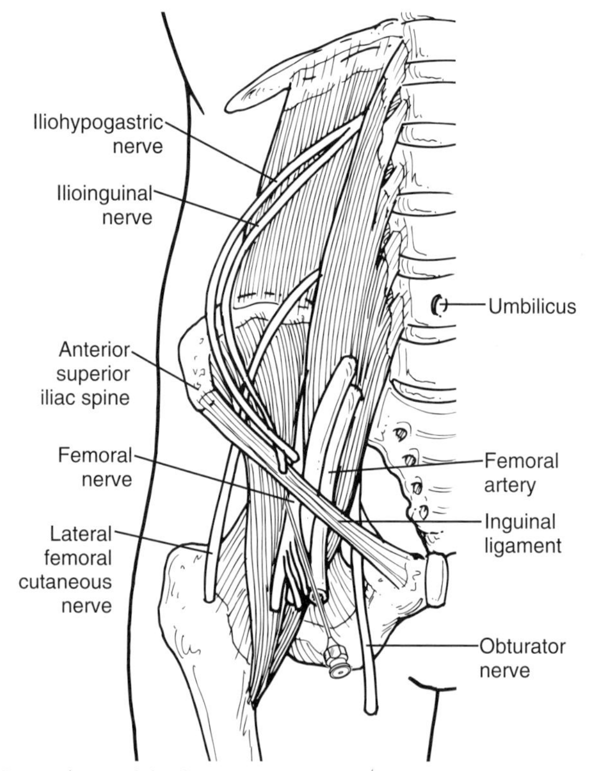

Fig 6–25 Femoral nerve injection.

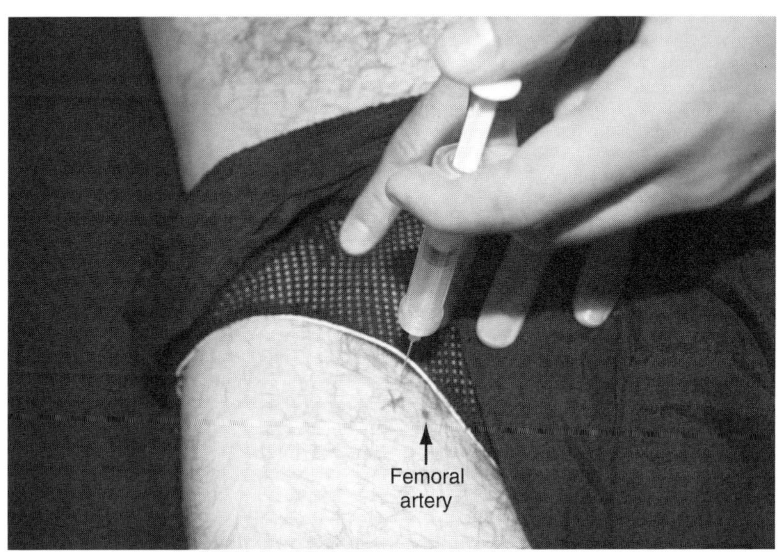

Fig 6–26 Femoral nerve injection.

nerve—withdraw the needle slightly. Do not inject forcefully because it is a fixed space and nerve trauma may result. Inject slowly.

Pitfalls/Complications

The patient may experience persistent paresthesia secondary to needle trauma to the nerve. The femoral artery and vein are located close to the injection site. Avoid local anesthetic toxicity by injecting slowly and aspirating after each 5 mL. Intravascular injection can be avoided by aspirating before injecting. Apply pressure to the injection site after needle insertion. If there is no relief from the injection, consider other sources of pain (femoral neuropathy, lumbosacral radiculopathy, lumbar plexopathy). The risk of infection can be minimized with sterile preparation of the area and aseptic technique.

Postinjection Care

Apply pressure over the injection site. Have the patient ice the affected area for 20 minutes two to three times daily for the first 24–48 hours. Then begin local heat and gentle stretching exercises several days after the injection. Avoid vigorous exercise or running for several days.

When to Perform Follow-Up Injections

Although there are no strict guidelines, a reasonable approach is to reinject in 4–6 weeks if symptoms persist or return. Partial relief of symptoms is an indication for a repeat injection. Do not inject more than once per visit because warning paresthesias may not present immediately. A total of three injections in a given 12-month period is the accepted standard.

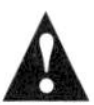

Saphenous Nerve Block

Name of Procedure

The name of this procedure is saphenous nerve block.

CPT

The Current Procedural Terminology code is unilateral 64450 (anesthetic agent—peripheral nerve).

Indications

This injection can be both diagnostic and therapeutic. This nerve can be blocked at either the medial aspect of the knee or the ankle. It can be blocked alone or with other nerves as anesthesia for surgical procedures of the foot. It can also be used to treat medial knee, medial leg, or foot pain when it is believed that the pain is due to entrapment or irritation of the saphenous nerve. A diagnostic saphenous nerve block may be helpful in distinguishing other causes of medial leg pain.

Symptoms

- Pain or paresthesias in the saphenous nerve distribution (medial knee pain, medial leg pain, or medial ankle and foot pain).
- Pain may only occur or may be exacerbated by sitting or squatting.

Physical Examination Findings

- Examination may be unremarkable.
- Tinel's sign may be present at the medial femoral condyle.
- Tinel's sign may also be present as the saphenous nerve crosses the ankle just anterior to the medial malleolus.
- Sensory deficits in the saphenous distribution may be present.
- Weakness should not be present (because this is a purely sensory nerve).
- Ankle reflexes and straight-leg raising should be normal.

Medications to Inject

A lidocaine/corticosteroid solution is injected for a therapeutic block, and lidocaine alone is injected for a diagnostic block.

Amount to Inject

The injectate amount is 4–7 mL.

Size and Gauge of Needle

A $\frac{5}{8}$-inch 25-gauge needle is used.

Local Anatomy

The saphenous nerve is a sensory branch of the femoral nerve. Its fibers originate at the L3, L4 nerve roots and travel through the lumbar plexus. In the thigh, the nerve travels with the femoral artery and become superficial in the medial distal thigh. The nerve crosses the medial femoral condyle between the tendons of the sartorius and the gracilis muscles. The nerve travels through the medial aspect of the lower leg and crosses the ankle anterior to the medial malleolus and medial to the tibialis anterior tendon. The saphenous nerve supplies sensation to the medial aspect of the knee, leg, ankle, and foot.

Patient Position

For saphenous nerve injection at the ankle injection, the patient should be lying prone. For injection at the knee, the patient lies prone with the leg slightly externally rotated or lies on the side with the medial knee of the affected leg exposed.

How and Where to Inject

The saphenous nerve can be blocked at the medial femoral condyle or at the ankle (Figures 6–27 and 6–28).

At the Level of the Knee

The medial femoral condyle is palpated. At the medial aspect of the medial condyle, the needle is advanced until either contact with the bone or paresthesias occur. At this point, the needle is slightly withdrawn, and approximately 5 mL of solution can be injected. This is a superficial injection with a needle depth of approximately ¼–½ inch. Because the saphenous vessels are quite close to this area, care should be taken to avoid intravascular injection (frequent aspiration with any needle repositioning).

At the Level of the Ankle

The anterior aspect of the medial malleolus and the tibialis anterior tendon as it crosses the ankle are the two main landmarks. The nerve lies anterior to the medial malleolus and medial to the tibialis anterior tendon. If the nerve is contacted or paresthesias are obtained, the needle should be withdrawn slightly. This is also a superficial injection (depth approximately ¼ inch). Approximately 5 mL of solution can be injected.

Pitfalls/Complications

Intraneural and intravascular injections are the primary complications. A postinjection hematoma or ecchymoses is not uncommon, and postinjection pressure along with ice can minimize associated pain and discomfort. The patient should be warned that the foot may

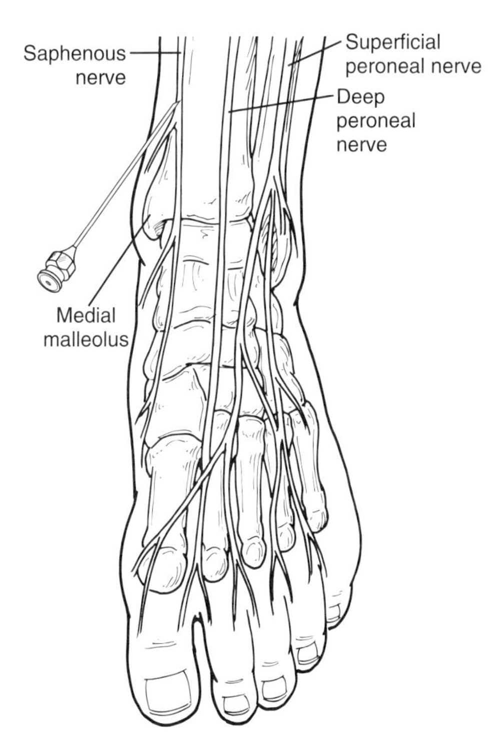

Fig 6–27 Saphenous nerve injection at ankle.

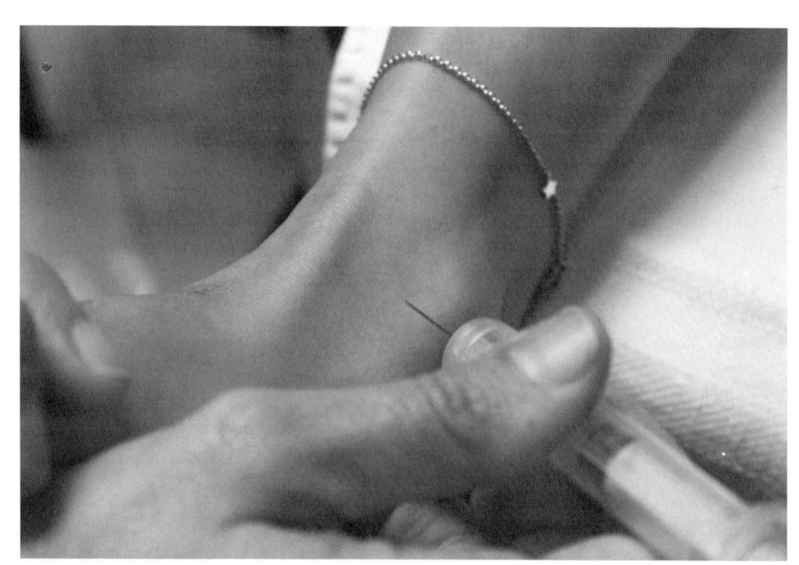

Fig 6–28 Saphenous nerve injection at ankle.

be insensate for a period of time and that walking on the foot during the period of anesthesia should be avoided. If there is no relief from the injection, consider other sources of pain (radiculopathy, plexopathy, femoral neuropathy at a more proximal location, peripheral neuropathy, or medial knee or ankle pain caused by articular or musculotendinous causes).

Postinjection Care

Apply pressure and ice (optional) over the injection site. Avoid vigorous exercise for several days. The patient should be prepared for a nerve anesthesia after injection.

When to Perform Follow-Up Injections

If the injection failed to elicit anesthesia, a repeat injection should be performed. The length of response to a successful injection and whether the injection was diagnostic or therapeutic will dictate the need for further injections.

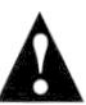

Tibial Nerve Injection (Tarsal Tunnel Injection)

Name of Procedure

The name of this procedure is tibial nerve block.

CPT

The Current Procedural Terminology code is unilateral 64450 (anesthetic agent—peripheral nerve) and neurolytic 64640 (pheno neurolysis—peripheral nerve).

Indications

The indication for this injection is tarsal tunnel syndrome. This injection can be both diagnostic and therapeutic. Injection is usually done after the patient has had a course of NSAIDs, physical therapy modalities and stretching, medial arch support, foot orthosis, or a short leg-walking cast fail. Electrodiagnostic testing may be very helpful in the diagnosis of tarsal tunnel syndrome, as well as in localizing a lesion to individual branches.

Symptoms

- Foot pain and paresthesia, frequently aggravated by prolonged walking.
- Symptoms may radiate to the calf.
- Depending on which branch of the tibial nerve is compressed, symptoms may vary.
- Heel pain.

Physical Examination Findings

- Sensory deficits or paresthesia in a posterior tibial nerve distribution.
- A Tinel's sign may be present over the posterior tibial nerve behind the medial malleolus.
- Symptoms may be reproduced with great toe extension or sustained passive ankle eversion.
- Foot muscle atrophy may be present.

Medications to Inject

A local anesthetic/corticosteroid solution is injected.

Amount to Inject

The injectate amount is 5–7 mL.

Size and Gauge of Needle

A 1½-inch 25-gauge needle is used.

Local Anatomy

The tibial nerve travels under the flexor retinaculum, which lies between the medial malleolus and the Achilles tendon. The tibial artery and vein, as well as the tibialis posterior and the flexor digitorum tendons, also travel in this space. The tibial nerve runs posterior to the tibial artery. The tibial nerve divides into its two main branches in the region of the tarsal tunnel. These branches are the medial plantar nerve and the lateral plantar nerve. The medial calcaneal nerve generally branches off the tibial nerve at or above the tarsal tunnel and supplies sensation to the medial and plantar surfaces of the heel. The medial plantar nerve supplies sensation to the medial 2–3 toes on the surface of the foot. The first branch of the lateral plantar nerve supplies the abductor digiti quinti muscle. It is also called the inferior calcaneal nerve or Baxter's nerve. Entrapment of this branch is thought by some to be a cause of intractable heel pain. The lateral plantar nerve supplies sensation to the lateral 2–3 toes on the plantar surface of the foot.

Patient Position

The patient lies on his/her side with the medial ankle of the involved leg facing upward.

How and Where to Inject

Palpate the tibial artery between the medial malleolus and the Achilles tendon (Figures 6–29 and 6–30). After sterile preparation and with aseptic technique, the needle should be inserted just posterior to the tibial artery and angled slightly anteriorly. The needle should be inserted approximately 1–2 cm. At this point, the needle tip

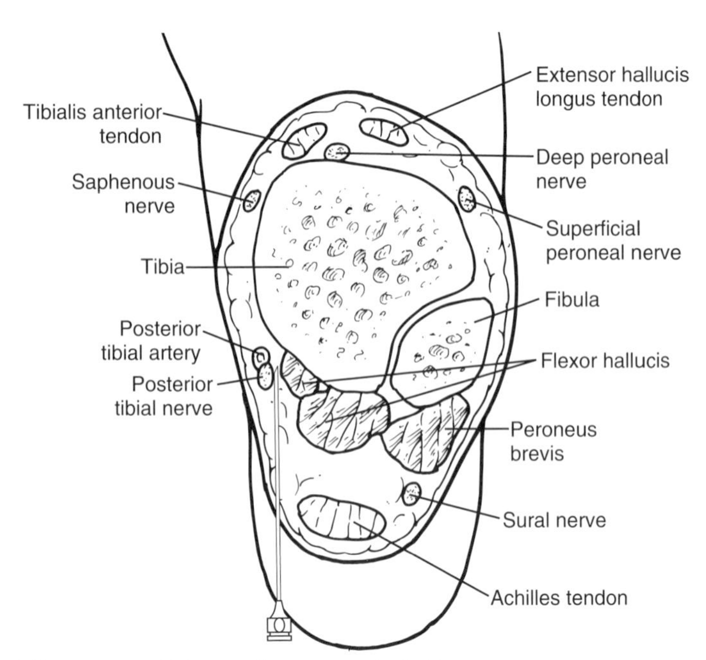

Fig 6–29 Posterior tibial nerve (tarsal tunnel) injection.

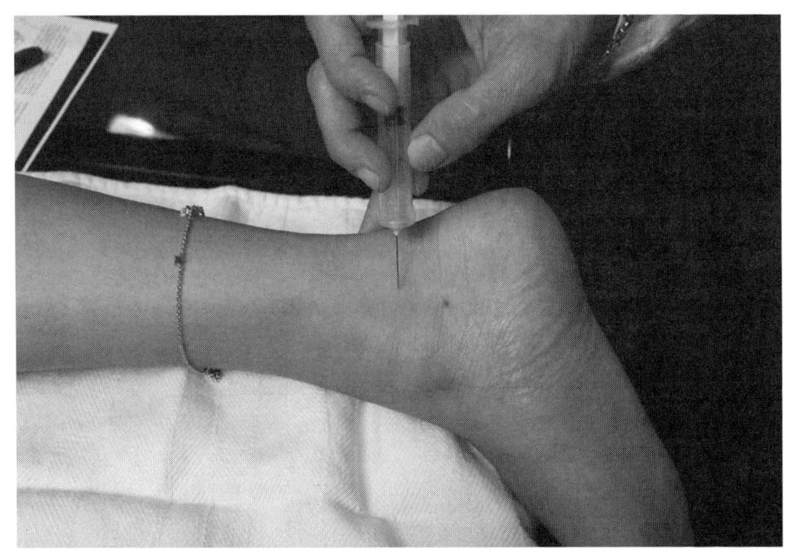

Fig 6–30 Posterior tibial nerve (tarsal tunnel) injection.

should be in the tarsal tunnel and in close proximity to the tibial nerve. Care should be taken to avoid intraneural injection. If paresthesia is elicited (the patient should be warned of this possibility), the needle should be withdrawn slightly. Aspirate before injecting to ensure the needle has not entered a vascular structure. Some physicians use a nerve stimulator to help localize the nerve.

Pitfalls/Complications

The patient should be warned of postinjection anesthesia in the foot after injection. Weightbearing should be minimized during this time. Given the close proximity of blood vessels to the nerve, ecchymoses and/or hematoma are possible. This can be minimized by postinjection compression. If the tibial artery is entered, the injection should be discontinued and pressure maintained to minimize hematoma. If there is no relief from the injection, consider other sources of pain (lumbar radiculopathy, complex regional pain syndrome, peripheral neuropathy, tibial nerve entrapment proximal to the tarsal tunnel, posterior tibial tendinitis, arthritis of the subtalar joint, plantar fasciitis, and lumbosacral plexopathy).

Postinjection Care

Apply pressure and ice over the injection site. Avoid vigorous exercise for several days. The patient should be prepared for a nerve anesthesia after injection.

When to Perform Follow-Up Injections

If anesthesia was not achieved, the injection was likely not in the region of the tibial nerve, and repeat injection should be considered. If anesthesia was achieved but the symptoms persist, a diagnosis other than tarsal tunnel syndrome should be considered. No hard guidelines exist, but a limit of three injections is probably prudent. Surgery can be considered in cases not responding to conservative management or injection therapy.

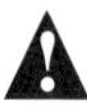

Deep Peroneal Nerve Injection (Anterior Tarsal Tunnel)

Name of Procedure

The name of this procedure is deep peroneal nerve block in the anterior tarsal tunnel.

CPT

The Current Procedural Terminology code is unilateral 64550 (anesthetic agent—peripheral nerve).

Indications

The indication for this injection is anterior foot pain. This injection can be both diagnostic and therapeutic. Entrapment or irritation of the deep peroneal nerve as it crosses the ankle can be due to trauma (most commonly tight shoes) or stretching against the extensor retinaculum. Electrodiagnostic testing may show an increased distal peroneal motor latency compared with the opposite side.

Symptoms

- Paresthesias or dysesthesias in the first web space (the skin supplied by this nerve).
- In severe lesions, weakness of the extensor digitorum brevis (EDB) muscle may be noted.

Physical Examination Findings

- Unlikely to show evidence of weakness.
- Weakness of peroneal innervated muscles other than the EDB suggests a more proximal lesion.

- Sensory deficits or paresthesias, if present, should be in a deep peroneal distribution (the first web space on the dorsum of the foot).
- A Tinel's sign may be present in the anterior ankle just medial to the extensor hallucis longus (EHL).

Medications to Inject

A local anesthetic/corticosteroid solution is injected.

Amount to Inject

The injectate amount is 5–7 mL.

Size and Gauge of Needle

A 1½-inch 25-gauge needle is used.

Local Anatomy

The deep and superficial peroneal nerves are the terminal branches of the common peroneal nerve. Just above the knee, the sciatic nerve divides into its two main terminal branches (the tibial and peroneal nerves). In the popliteal fossa, the common peroneal nerve is more lateral than the tibial nerve and travels just behind the fibular head. Below the fibula, the nerve divides into the deep and superficial branches. The only muscles supplied by the superficial branch are the peroneus longus and brevis. The superficial peroneal nerve crosses the anterolateral ankle superficial to the flexor retinaculum and supplies sensation to the dorsum of the foot with the exception of the first web space.

The deep peroneal nerve supplies all of the muscles in the anterior compartment of the leg with the exception of the peroneus longus and brevis. It also supplies the extensor digitorum brevis (EDB) in the foot. The deep peroneal nerve crosses the ankle just medial to the extensor hallucis longus (EHL) beneath the extensor retinaculum. It supplies sensation on the dorsum of the foot between the first two toes (the first dorsal web space).

Patient Position

The patient is supine with the anterior ankle exposed.

How and Where to Inject

The EHL should be identified at the level of the malleoli (Figures 6–31 and 6–32). This can be accomplished by having the patient extend only the great toe. The dorsalis pedis artery should also be identified. Injection should be just medial to the EHL tendon. The nerve is deep to the extensor retinaculum. If paresthesia is elicited (the patient should be warned of this possibility), the needle should be withdrawn slightly. Aspirate before injecting to ensure the needle has not entered a vascular structure (dorsalis pedis artery).

Pitfalls/Complications

The patient should be warned of a period of anesthesia in the foot after injection. Weight-bearing should be minimized during this time. Given the close proximity of blood vessels to the nerve, ecchymosis and/or hematomas are possible. This can be minimized by postinjection compression. If there is no relief from the injection, consider other sources of pain (lumbar radiculopathy, peripheral neuropathy, sciatic neuropathy, common peroneal neuropathy, more proximal deep peroneal neuropathy, superficial peroneal neuropathy and lumbar plexopathy).

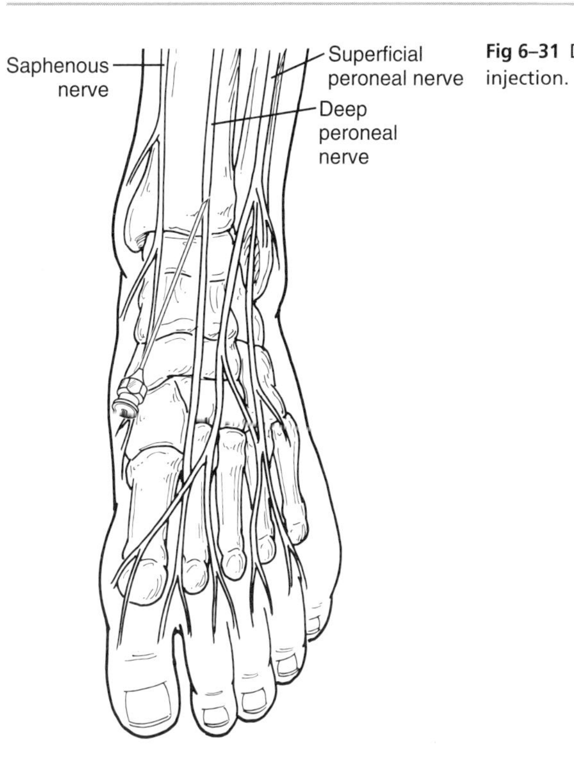

Fig 6–31 Deep peroneal nerve injection.

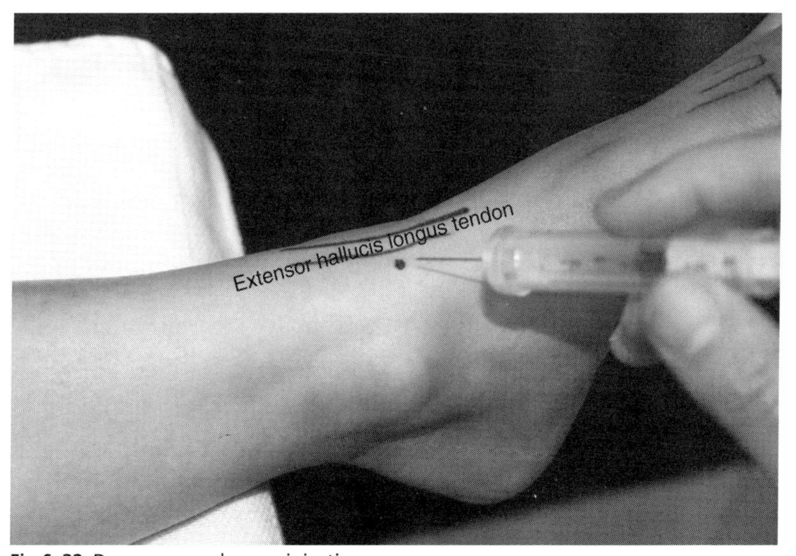

Fig 6–32 Deep peroneal nerve injection.

Postinjection Care

Apply pressure and ice over the injection site. Avoid vigorous exercise for several days. The patient should be prepared for a nerve anesthesia after injection.

When to Perform Follow-Up Injections

If anesthesia was not achieved, the injection was likely not in the region of the deep peroneal nerve, and repeat injection should be considered. If anesthesia was achieved but the symptoms persisted, another diagnosis should be considered. No hard guidelines exist, but a limit of three injections is probably prudent.

Superficial Peroneal—Nerve Injection at the Ankle

Name of Procedure

The name of this procedure is superficial peroneal nerve block.

CPT

The Current Procedural Terminology code is unilateral 64550 (anesthetic agent—peripheral nerve).

Indications

The indication for this procedure is anterior foot pain. This injection can be both diagnostic and therapeutic. Paresthesias in the distribution of the superficial peroneal nerve may be due to irritation or entrapment of this nerve at the ankle. Because this nerve generally is superficial to the extensor retinaculum, entrapment at this level is less likely than the deep peroneal nerve. The nerve can, however, be compressed by tight shoes. Electrodiagnostic testing is unlikely to be helpful in diagnosing a superficial peroneal neuropathy. It can, however, be very helpful in excluding a deep peroneal neuropathy or a more proximal superficial or common peroneal neuropathy. It can also be helpful in determining whether symptoms are due to a radiculopathy or sciatic nerve entrapment.

Symptoms

- Paresthesias in the distribution of the superficial peroneal nerve.
- Because this nerve has no motor innervation below the ankle, weakness suggests a more proximal entrapment.

Physical Examination Findings

- Should not show evidence of weakness. (Weakness of the extensor digitorum brevis [EDB] or other peroneal innervation muscles suggests a more proximal lesion or a deep peroneal nerve lesion.)
- Sensory deficits or paresthesia, if present, should be in a superficial peroneal distribution (the dorsum of the foot sparing the first web space).
- A Tinel's sign may be present in the anterolateral ankle lateral to the extensor hallucis longus (EHL).

Medications to Inject

A local anesthetic solution, usually without epinephrine, is injected. Because this is a very superficial injection, the initial block should be diagnostic and consist only of local anesthetic. If sufficient pain relief is obtained after one or more diagnostic blocks, an injection with corticosteroid can be considered.

Amount to Inject

The injectate amount is 5–7 mL.

Size and Gauge of Needle

A 1-inch 25-gauge needle is used.

Local Anatomy

The deep and superficial peroneal nerves are the terminal branches of the common peroneal nerve. Just above the knee, the sciatic nerve divides into its two main terminal branches (the tibial and peroneal nerves). The common peroneal nerve is more lateral than the tibial nerve in the popliteal fossa, and it travels just behind the fibular head. Below the fibula, the nerve divides into the deep and superficial branches. The only muscles supplied by the superficial branch are the peroneus longus and brevis. This nerve then crosses the anterolateral ankle superficial to the extensor retinaculum. It supplies sensation to the dorsum of the foot with the exception of the first web space (which is supplied by the deep branch).

Patient Position

The patient lies supine with the anterior ankle exposed.

How and Where to Inject

Because the superficial peroneal nerve has divided into several branches at the level of the anterior ankle, the subcutaneous region needs to be infiltrated (Figures 6–33 and 6–34). The injection is in the anterolateral ankle at the level of the intermalleolar line. It should

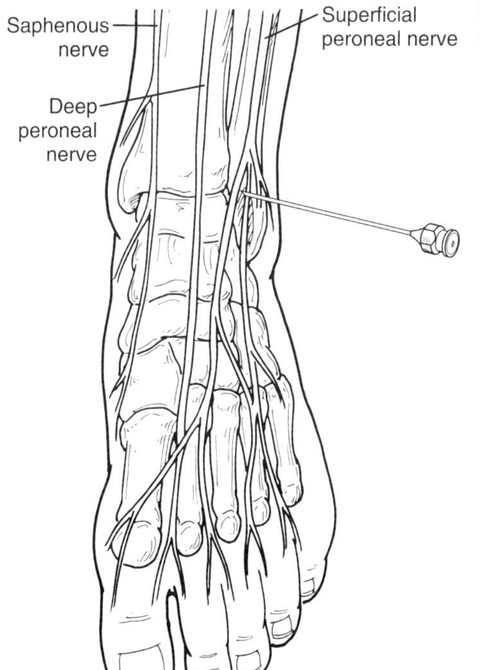

Fig 6–33 Superficial peroneal nerve injection.

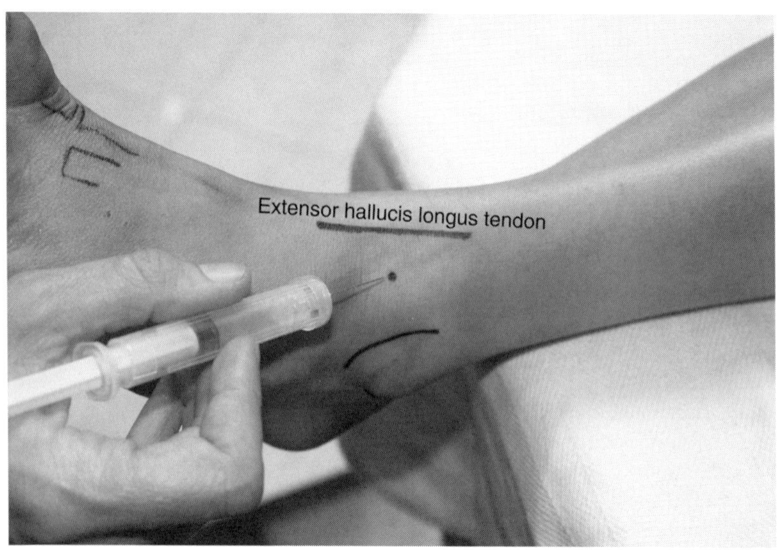

Fig 6–34 Superficial peroneal nerve injection.

be lateral to the extensor hallucis longus (EHL) tendon and anterior to the fibula. Care should be taken to avoid intraneural injection. If paresthesia is elicited (the patient should be warned of this possibility), the needle should be withdrawn slightly. Aspirate before injecting to ensure the needle has not entered a vascular structure.

Pitfalls/Complications

The patient should be warned of a period of anesthesia in the foot after injection. Weight-bearing should be minimized during this time. Because of the superficial nature of this block, the patient should be aware of the likelihood of skin discoloration with corticosteroid use. If there is no relief from the injection, consider other sources of pain (lumbar radiculopathy, peripheral neuropathy, sciatic neuropathy, common peroneal neuropathy, deep peroneal neuropathy, more proximal superficial peroneal neuropathy and lumbar plexopathy).

Postinjection Care

Apply pressure and ice over the injection site. Avoid vigorous exercise for several days. The patient should be prepared for a nerve anesthesia after injection.

When to Perform Follow-Up Injections

If anesthesia was not achieved, the injection was likely not in the region of the superficial peroneal nerve, and repeat injection should be considered. If anesthesia was achieved but the symptoms persist, another diagnosis should be considered. If sufficient pain relief is obtained after one or more diagnostic blocks, an injection with corticosteroid can be considered. No hard guidelines exist, but a limit of three injections is probably prudent.

Sural Nerve Block

Name of Procedure

The name of this procedure is sural nerve block.

CPT

The Current Procedural Terminology code is unilateral 64450 (anesthetic agent—peripheral nerve).

Indications

This injection can be both diagnostic and therapeutic. Although the sural nerve is most commonly blocked for local anesthesia, a block may have implications in diagnosing and treating pain syndromes.

Symptoms

- Pain or paresthesias in the sural nerve distribution.

Physical Examination Findings

- Examination may be unremarkable.
- Sensation in the foot (sural nerve distribution) may be diminished. The sensory examination should try to distinguish between a sural nerve lesion (affecting sensation to the posterolateral aspect of the calf and the lateral aspect of the foot) and an S1 radiculopathy (which would affect the posterior thigh as well).
- Ankle reflexes and straight-leg raising should be normal.

Medications to Inject

A lidocaine/corticosteroid solution should be injected for a therapeutic block, and lidocaine alone should be injected for a diagnostic block.

Amount to Inject

The injectate amount is 5–10 mL.

Size and Gauge of Needle

A 1-inch 25-gauge needle is used.

Local Anatomy

The sural nerve receives its innervation from the lumbosacral plexus (L5, S1). In the posterior thigh, the sciatic nerve divides into its two main branches: the common peroneal nerve and the tibial nerve. Each of these nerves gives off a branch, which together forms the sural nerve. This nerve arises below the knee and travels superficially in the posterior leg. The nerve is located near the midline in the lower leg and travels behind the lateral malleolus to innervate the foot. The sural nerve supplies sensation to the posterolateral aspect of the calf and the lateral aspect of the foot.

Patient Position

The patient lies prone.

How and Where to Inject

The sural nerve is most easily blocked at the level of the lateral malleolus (Figures 6–35 and 6–36). The needle is inserted in the midpoint between the Achilles tendon and the lateral malleolus. If paresthesias are obtained, the needle should be slightly repositioned (to avoid an intraneural injection) and the medication injected. Anesthesia in a sural distribution confirms a successful block. Aspirate before injecting to avoid intravascular administration.

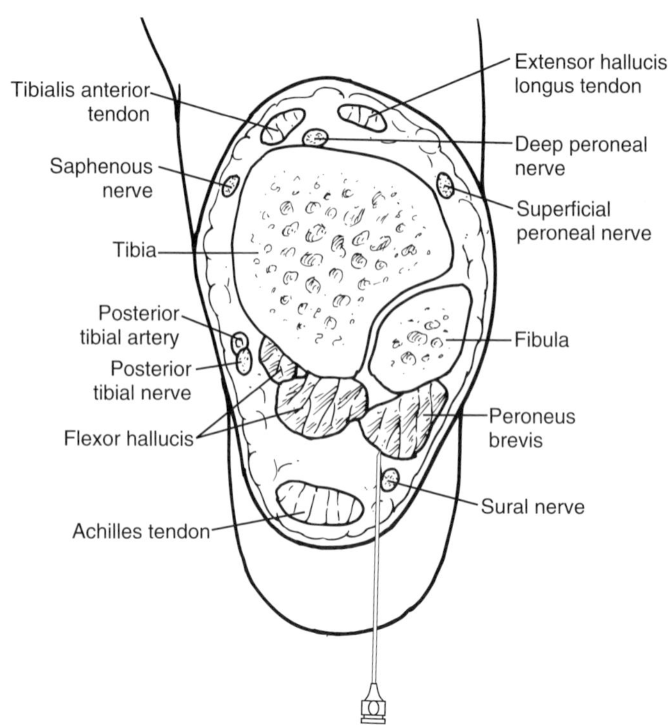

Fig 6–35 Sural nerve injection.

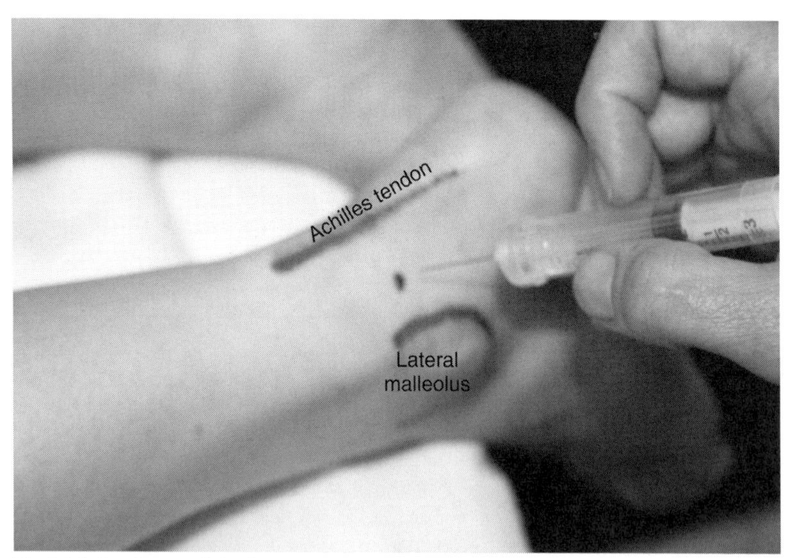

Fig 6–36 Sural nerve injection.

Pitfalls/Complications

Intraneural and intravascular injections are the primary complications. The patient should be warned that the foot may be insensate for a period of time and that walking on the foot during the period of anesthesia should be avoided. If there is no relief from the injection, consider other sources of pain (lumbar radiculopathy, peripheral neuropathy, sciatic neuropathy, tibial neuropathy, peroneal neuropathy, and lumbar plexopathy).

Postinjection Care

Apply pressure and ice (optional) over the injection site. Avoid vigorous exercise for several days. The patient should be prepared for a nerve anesthesia after injection.

When to Perform Follow-Up Injections

If the injection failed to elicit anesthesia, a repeat injection should be performed. The length of response to a successful injection and whether the injection was diagnostic or therapeutic will dictate the need for further injections.

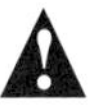

Lower Extremity Digital Nerve Blocks

Name of Procedure

The name of this procedure is interdigital nerve block.

CPT

The Current Procedural Terminology code is 64450 (anesthetic agent—peripheral nerve).

Indications

These injections are most often used for local anesthesia. In pain syndromes, these injections can be helpful in the treatment of interdigital neuromas (Morton's neuroma).

Symptoms

- Morton's neuroma is manifested by foot pain localized to the interdigital space.
- Pain can extend to the toes.

Physical Examination Findings

- Foot pain aggravated by mediolateral compression of the toes.

Medications to Inject

Local anesthetics are injected only for nerve block (local anesthetics with epinephrine are absolutely contraindicated in interdigital or digital injections). Local anesthetic with corticosteroid is used for neuroma injections.

Amount to Inject

The injectate amount is 2–3 cc.

Size and Gauge of Needle

A 1½-inch 25-gauge needle is used.

Local Anatomy

The tibial nerve (posterior tibial nerve) travels behind in the medial malleolus of the ankle. The tibial nerve generally has four terminal branches that are given off at approximately the level of the ankle. The final two branches are the medial and lateral plantar nerves. These nerves innervate the intrinsic foot muscles. The terminal branches of these nerves become the interdigital nerves, supplying sensation to the toes. As the name implies, the interdigital nerves travel between the two digits that they supply. The nerve divides about the level of the metatarsal head. The branches supply the medial surface of one toe and the lateral surface of the adjoining toe.

How and Where to Inject

The needle should be inserted on the dorsal surface of the foot, between the adjoining metatarsal heads (Figures 6–37 and 6–38). The patient should be warned in advance to

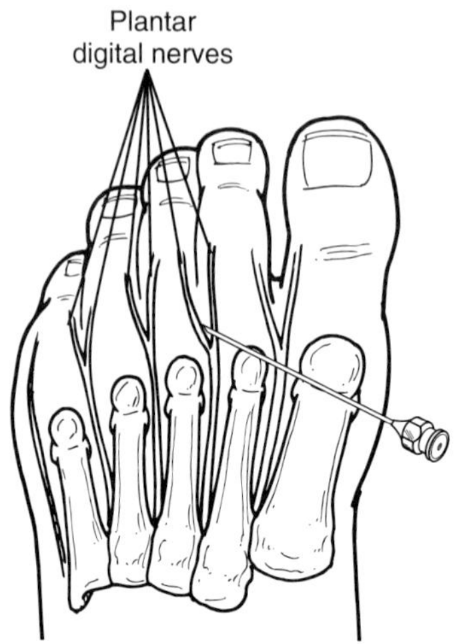

Fig 6–37 Lower extremity digital nerve injection.

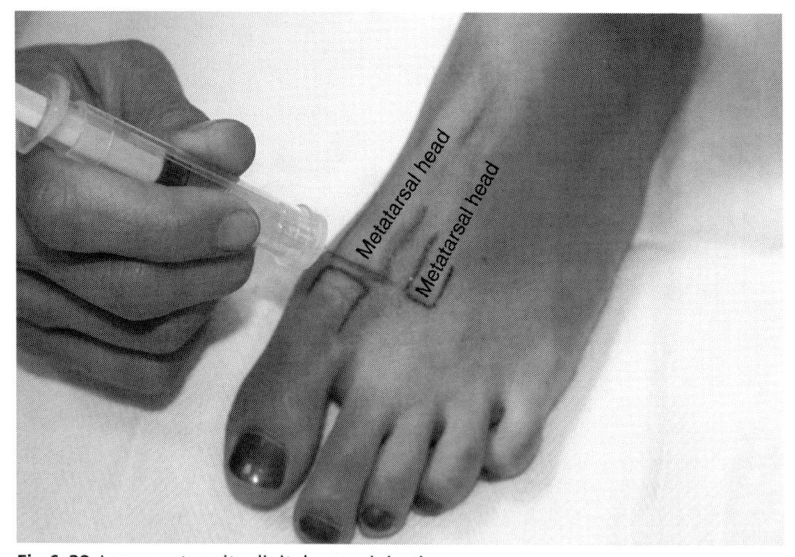

Fig 6–38 Lower extremity digital nerve injection.

notify the physician if paresthesias are felt. The needle is advanced 1½–2 cm. Postinjection anesthesia of the adjoining surfaces of two toes will confirm the injection was in the proper area. Aspirate before injecting to avoid intravascular administration.

Pitfalls/Complications

The patient may experience paresthesias secondary to needle trauma of the nerve. A hematoma also may occur, causing localized pain and pressure on the nerve. The risk of infection can be minimized with sterile preparation of the area and aseptic technique.

Postinjection Care

Apply pressure over the injection site. Use ice on the affected area for 20 minutes two to three times a day for the first day. Have the patient avoid excessive walking, and essentially treat the foot as an insensate foot until the local anesthetic wears off.

When to Perform Follow-Up Injections

Although there are no strict guidelines, a reasonable approach is to reinject in 4–6 weeks if symptoms persist or return. Partial relief of symptoms is an indication for a repeat injection. Do not inject more than once per visit because warning paresthesias may not be present in subsequent injections. A total of three injections in a given 12-month period is the generally accepted standard.

7

Trigger Point Injections

In myofascial pain problems, there are frequently trigger and/or tender points that are characterized by exquisitely sensitive areas in the soft tissues. These are often "knotty" areas of the muscle. Trigger points are described as discrete, focal, hyperirritable spots that are usually located in a taut band of muscle but may be found in ligaments, periosteum, tendons, and pericapsular areas (Alvarez and Rockwell, 2002). Trigger points are called such because they trigger or refer pain into a specific distant area called a "reference pain zone." The referred pain from trigger points is generally predictable, and these patterns are "mapped" in trigger point manuals.

Trigger points may be classified as active or latent. Active trigger points cause pain at rest, whereas latent ones do not cause spontaneous pain but may restrict movement or cause muscle weakness (Fisher, 2000). Often, latent trigger points are only identified when an examiner places direct pressure over the site. In many instances when firm pressure is applied to a trigger point, there is a local twitch response in which the muscle spontaneously contracts. This may also occur when the region comes into contact with a needle. Tender points are associated only with pain at the site of palpation and do not have referred pain or a local twitch response.

It is not known why some people develop trigger points; however, it is likely that acute trauma or repetitive microtrauma plays a role. Factors that may contribute to the development of trigger points may also include lack of exercise, poor posture, vitamin deficiencies, sleep disturbances, and structural support issues such as joint problems.

Injections are often a reasonable way to treat trigger points and often work quite well. They may be used as a first-line intervention; however, many practitioners prefer to try other methods first. Some of the treatment interventions one could try include acupuncture or acupressure, osteopathic manual medicine techniques, massage, deep heat with ultrasound, superficial application of heat or ice, diathermy, transcutaneous electrical nerve stimulation (TENS), and Spray and Stretch technique (applying dichlorodifluoromethane-trichloromonofluoromethane [Fluori-Methane] or ethyl chloride spray topically).

Mechanism of Action

Trigger point injections can be done in a variety of different ways, which often depends on the skill, training, and preference of the practitioner. For example, local anesthetic may be injected alone or with corticosteroid. Some practitioners will use sterile saline, particularly if there is a history of an allergy to "caine" medications. Although the medications can provide short-term relief, the key to success in relieving pain seems to be from the mechanical effects of the needling itself (Fisher, 2000). This seems to break up the abnormal tissue. This is why some practitioners prefer to simply perform a "dry needling" technique that does not involve using any medications.

Typically, one or two areas are injected during a single office visit. Several injections may be done, depending on the patient's tolerance. This procedure may be repeated every few days for acute pain. Once the pain is better controlled, the time between injections can be spread out or the procedure discontinued altogether.

Potential Risks

The risks associated with trigger point injections are somewhat similar to botulinum toxin risks. However, there seems to be an increased concern with muscle injury when trigger point injections are performed with local anesthetics or corticosteroids. As with botulinum toxin injections, the risks fall into categories that include:

1. Reactions to the medication(s).
2. Overdosing.
3. Poor injection technique.

Reactions to the Medication(s) and Overdosing

Although trigger point injections are generally thought to be safe when done by experienced practitioners, local anesthetics and corticosteroids are known to cause reactions at the muscular level that may result in myotoxicity. Injury to the muscle may depend on the medication, dose, volume, and number of times the injection is repeated (e.g., serial injections may lead to myotoxicity) (Zink and Graf, 2004). In general, if you use medications with these injections, it is best to limit the dose and volume. Overdosing is particularly a concern with local anesthetics because the effects may spread to areas that are not involved or there may be a more generalized anesthetic effect that can impact respiratory function and so forth. Refer to the example for suggested techniques and doses.

Poor Injection Technique

Poor injection technique may result in significant complications such as pneumothorax, injury to a blood vessel or nerve, or damage to a vital organ. Once again, expert knowledge of the anatomy is essential to safely perform these injections.

Trigger point injections are a relatively safe and easy office procedure that can markedly alleviate myofascial pain. Although these injections can be used as a first-line treatment, it is best to not overuse them, especially if local anesthetics or corticosteroids are being used. Also, relief may be more effective and prolonged if these are done in conjunction with other treatments such as oral muscle relaxants and physical therapy.

Name of Procedure

The name for this procedure is a trigger point injection.

CPT

The Current Procedural Terminology codes are 20552 (two muscle group) and 20553 (three muscle group).

Indications

The indication for this injection is a muscularly related pain problem. This may be an appropriate first-line treatment for acute muscular injuries or more chronic conditions such as fibromyalgia. Trigger point injections work best if the pain is confined regionally (diffuse and widespread pain is not usually an indication for these injections).

Symptoms

- Myofascial regional or localized pain.

Physical Examination Findings

- Pain with direct palpation to the affected area.
- Radiating pain to specific regions associated with the trigger point.
- Palpable taut band.
- Local twitch response may be present.

Medications to Inject

We recommend either dry needling (with no medication) or the use of a small amount of local anesthetic. Occasionally, practitioners will use saline, especially if there is a "caine" allergy. Examples of appropriate local anesthetics include 1% lidocaine or 0.5% procaine.

Amount to Inject

We recommend that the amount of local anesthetic injected be limited. A reasonable amount is 0.1–0.3 mL each time you stop the needle penetration. The total volume injected will depend on how many injections you perform. Usually, the total amount is in the range of 1–12 mL.

Size and Gauge of Needle

A 22- to 25-gauge needle is recommended. The length of the needle depends on the depth you are aiming to achieve. You want your needle to be longer than the depth of the entire trigger point, although you have to be careful about underlying structures when injecting.

Local Anatomy

The trigger point to be injected should be superficial and easily accessible.

Patient Position

Have the patient lie down (prone or supine) if possible. Injections may be done in a seated position as well.

How and Where to Inject

For myofascial, pain it is best to inject into the tender/trigger point, hopefully eliciting a local twitch response (Figure 7–1). To provide optimal patient comfort, spray the area first with a vapocoolant spray such as Fluoromethane. Then aim and insert the needle into the trigger point, and when you stop penetrating, draw back. If there is no blood, slowly inject 0.1–0.3 mL of your solution. Without removing the needle, reposition it within the trigger point and again draw back and inject if there is no aspirate. Typically, you will do this several times for each trigger point.

Pitfalls/Complications

Some people may complain of an increase in pain for a few days after the injection. Informing patients of this helps to alleviate their postinjection pain concerns. If there is

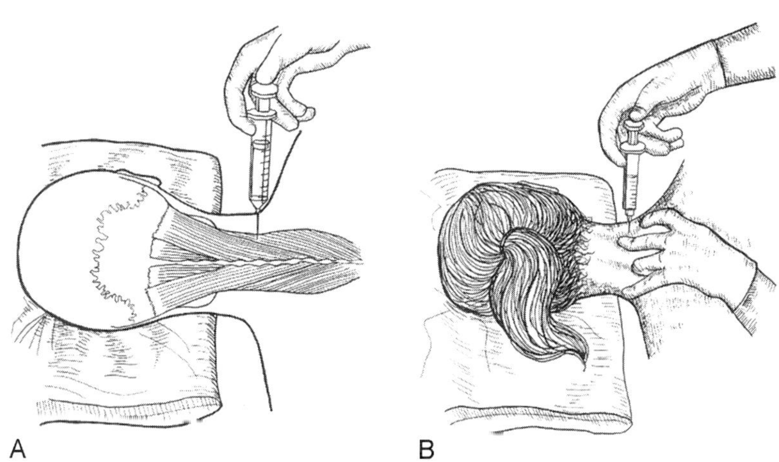

Fig 7–1 Injection of the lower trigger point area in the splenius cervicis muscle. (A) Location where the needle penetrates the muscle. (B) Injection of the trigger point as diagrammed in (A).

no relief or only partial pain relief, consider whether the injection reached the desired trigger point. Infection can usually be avoided by use of a sterile technique.

Postinjection Care

Apply pressure over the injection sites. Local heat may provide relief after the injection, although be sure that homeostasis has been achieved first. Gentle stretching exercises may be started several days after the injection. Avoid vigorous exercise in the affected area for several days. It is very important to tell patients to rest the affected area for the first couple of days after the injections.

When to Perform Follow-Up Injections

Although there are no strict guidelines, a reasonable approach is to reinject one to three times per week for acute pain. As the pain lessens, the length of time between injections can increase to once per week or even longer. For chronic pain conditions, trigger point injections are done on an as-needed basis. Some patients will require these only very infrequently (e.g., one to two times per year).

REFERENCES

Alvarez, D. J., and Rockwell, P. G. (2002). Trigger points: Diagnosis and management. *Am. Fam. Physician* **65,** 654.

Fisher, A. A. (2000). *In* Trigger Point Injection in Pain Procedures in Clinical Practice. (T. A. Lennard, Ed.). 2nd ed. pp. 153–154. Hanley and Belfus, Inc. Philadelphia, PA.

Zink, W., and Graf, B. M. (2004). Local anesthetic myotoxicity. *Regional Anesth. Pain Med.* **29,** 333–340.

8

Botulinum Toxin

In 1989, the Food and Drug Administration (FDA) licensed Botox® in the United States for the treatment of strabismus, essential blepharospasm, and hemifacial spasm (Chiders and Simons, 2000). All these ailments involve muscular control (rather than pain, per se), which is the mechanism by which botulinum toxin works. Since that time, both botulinum toxin A (Botox® available in the United States and Dysport® available in other countries such as the United Kingdom and New Zealand) and B (Myobloc®) have been studied for many different muscularly related pain conditions and other medical problems (refer to table). Although the FDA has not formally approved these drugs for the treatment of pain (as of the date of publication), they are frequently used "off-label," and the evidence is quite good that they work well in selected patients who have muscular pain complaints. For patients with dystonia or spasticity, botulinum toxin may be a first-line therapy. However, although botulinum toxin is becoming an increasingly accepted method of treating a variety of musculoskeletal pain conditions, it is worthwhile to remember that these are off-label uses, and this method of pain control should be tried when more conventional methods have failed.

Mechanism of Action

The term *botulinum toxin* actually describes several potent neural toxins that may cause paralysis, respiratory arrest, and even death when ingested. These toxins are produced by the bacteria *Clostridium botulinum*. Although it is lethal in its oral form, botulinum toxin is remarkably safe to use as an injection. Although there are actually seven distinct serotypes of botulinum toxin, only serotypes A and B are approved for use by the FDA. Botulinum toxin type A has been used clinically and in research studies far more than type B, although they both work well for pain.

When injected into muscle, botulinum toxin blocks the release of acetylcholine, a substance necessary for muscular contraction, at the neuromuscular junction. This produces a chemical denervation that results in a reduction of muscular contractions. In the first couple of days after injection, there is no clinical effect. Functional muscular weakness (localized paralysis) peaks at 2 weeks and lasts approximately 12 weeks. The amount of medication used typically depends on the size of the muscles being injected.

Generally, a practitioner will inject several areas of a muscle during a single office visit. This can be done with or without electromyography (EMG) guidance. EMG guidance is usually done to ensure that specific muscles are injected. This is particularly helpful in cases where the muscles to be injected are small or deep. Large superficial muscle injections do not typically need EMG guidance.

If the underlying condition remains unchanged (e.g., as is the case when treating wrinkles or movement disorders), the injection will need to be repeated. When botulinum toxin is used to treat muscular pain and spasm, however, a single set of injections might break the cycle and essentially produce a "cure." On the other hand, there are many pain conditions (e.g., migraines) that are ongoing, so repeated injections would be anticipated.

As with all injections, it is important to consider alternative interventions before considering botulinum toxin as an option. Moreover, it is also imperative to follow up with rehabilitative measures after a series of botulinum toxin injections. For example, measures such as supervised physical or occupational therapy, biofeedback, and oral pain medications may enhance the effects of the injection.

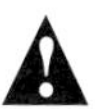

Potential Risks

Botulinum toxin is generally considered to have a wide safety margin (Naumann and Jankovic, 2004); however, there are inherent risks. The risks fall into three categories that include:

1. Reactions to the medication.
2. Overdosing.
3. Poor injection technique.

Reactions to the Medication

Allergic reactions to botulinum toxin are very rare. Botox hypersensitivity reactions have been reported to include anaphylaxis, urticaria, soft tissue edema, and dyspnea (Physicians' Desk Reference, 2005). One fatal case of Botox and lidocaine together was reported, although it is not certain which drug caused the reaction (Physician's Desk Reference, 2005). In individuals with preexisting neuromuscular disorders (e.g., amyotrophic lateral sclerosis, myasthenia gravis, and Eaton–Lambert syndrome), it is recommended that botulinum toxin be used with caution because there have been cases of systemic sensitivity with resultant dysphagia and respiratory compromise (Physician's Desk Reference, 2005). Dysphagia may also occur more locally when botulinum toxin is used in the paracervical region. In people who are taking aminoglycosides or other drugs that interfere with neuromuscular transmission (e.g., curare-like compounds), botulinum toxin should be used with caution because it may potentiate the effects of these drugs. Localized reactions may occur in the first 2 weeks and are similar to those of other injections, including pain, swelling, tenderness, and bruising at the injection site. These are usually transient and do not require medical intervention.

Overdosing

Because botulinum toxin causes functional weakness (you can think of this as a localized paralysis or partial paralysis of the injected muscle), it makes sense that injecting too much can "overparalyze" a region and lead to significant problems. Examples include the unintended paralysis of facial muscles, problems with dysphagia, and excessive limb weakness. Because the effects do wear off, this is not a permanent problem, but it can be quite debilitating during the time that the drug is in effect. A longer discussion with dosing recommendations can be found in Chapter 2.

Poor Injection Technique

Botulinum toxin should be delivered only to muscles; therefore, it is important to aspirate and be sure that you are not injecting into a blood vessel. Poor injection technique may lead to injury to an organ or nerve. Another technique problem occurs if the wrong muscle is injected and you do not get the desired effect. In addition, you may induce weakness in a muscle that you did not intend.

In general, botulinum toxin is a relatively safe and easy medication to inject. It can provide significant pain relief for many weeks to patients who are suffering. However, it should be considered only after conventional pain treatments have been tried and failed. Moreover, it is important to pay particular attention to dosing and ensure that you are injecting into the appropriate muscle.

Botulinum Toxin Clinical Uses (Allam *et al.*, 2005; Charles, 2004; Ghazizadeh and Nikzad, 2004; Childers and Simons, 2000; Thomson *et al.*, 2005)

- Anal fissure
- Anismus
- Cervical whiplash
- Detrusor-sphincter dyssynergia
- Dystonia (e.g., cervical/spasmodic torticollis, laryngeal/spasmodic dysphonia, and occupational/writer's cramp)
- Esophageal achalasia
- Essential blepharospasm
- Essential tremor
- Facial wrinkles
- Headaches (e.g., migraine, tension-type, and cervicogenic)
- Hemifacial spasm
- Hyperhydrosis
- Low back pain
- Muscle cramps/spasm
- Myoclonus
- Myofascial pain syndrome
- Myokymia
- Nystagmus
- Pelvic pain syndromes
- Piriformis syndrome
- Sialorrhea
- Spasticity
- Strabismus
- Tics
- Trigeminal neuralgia
- Vaginismus

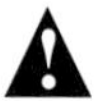

Injection Procedure

Name of Procedure

The name of the procedure is botulinum toxin injection.

CPT

The Current Procedural Terminology codes are 64612 (facial), 64613 (cervical), 64614 (extremity or trunk), and 95869 (EMG limited muscles one limb).

Indications

The indications for these injections are muscularly related pain problems, spasticity, or dystonia. This may be an appropriate first-line treatment for dystonia or spasticity; however, it is not a first-line treatment for pain and should be used only after other conventional treatments have been tried and failed. Often a local anesthetic injection is done as a "test" to determine whether botulinum toxin (which is longer acting) will be helpful. As a first-line agent, botulinum toxin may be particularly helpful when used for spasticity secondary to stroke, cerebral palsy, and so forth. If spasticity is impairing function or hygiene, injections can be therapeutic. It is ideal, although not necessary, if the spasticity is limited to one area. If there is more generalized spasticity, which is not amenable to systemic treatments alone, botulinum toxin may be tried.

Symptoms

- Muscular origin of pain.
- There may be associated spasticity, dystonia, or muscle spasm.
- Pain should be localized to a specific muscular region.

Physical Examination Findings

- Pain with direct palpation to the affected muscle(s).
- Reproduction of pain with certain movements that stress the muscle(s).
- It is common to have tender/trigger points, and there may be a local twitch response.

Medications to Inject

There are two commercially available botulinum toxin preparations in the United States. Botulinum toxin type A (Botox) and type B (Myobloc) have different dosing schedules and units, for one cannot be converted to the other.

Amount to Inject

It is important to refer to the manufacturers' suggested guidelines. The volume injected will depend on the size of the muscle and the dilution used.

Size and Gauge of Needle

A 2.5-inch 21-gauge needle is recommended for reconstitution (adding the botulinum toxin to the saline solution). For injection purposes, the needle size will vary depending on the muscle(s) to be injected. However, generally, a 25-, 27-, or 30-gauge needle is used for superficial muscles. A longer 22-gauge needle may be used for deeper musculature.

Local Anatomy

The muscle to be injected should be superficial and easily accessible, otherwise EMG guidance is indicated.

Patient Position

Have the patient lie down (prone or supine) if possible. Injections may be done in a seated position as well.

How and Where to Inject

For myofascial pain, it is best to inject into the tender/trigger point, hopefully eliciting a local twitch response (Figure 8–1). Typically, several injections are done during a single procedure. For spasticity, again several locations are typically injected. Many physicians prefer to use EMG guidance for this procedure; although if the muscle you are injecting is large and the location obvious and readily accessible, it is not necessary.

Pitfalls/Complications

It is anticipated that the patient may have an increase in pain for a few days because of the local injection and the fact that the botulinum toxin will not be effective until after the first 48 hours or so. Informing patients of this helps to alleviate their postinjection pain concerns. If there is no relief or only partial pain relief, consider whether the injection reached the desired muscle(s) and whether the dose was sufficient. Infection can usually be avoided by use of sterile technique. The patient should be notified that transient flulike symptoms might be noted several days after the injection. These symptoms usually resolve spontaneously. Headaches, weakness, and localized swelling have also been reported. Gradual intolerance to botulinum toxin caused by antibody formation has been reported. Because botulinum toxin is a neurotoxin, the potential for fatal overdosing remains a possibility. However, if suggested dose regimens are followed, the likelihood of this is extremely low. The lethal dose of botulinum toxin A is 40 units/kg or approximately 3000 units for a 70-kg man. The normal dosing is less than $\frac{1}{10}$ this amount.

Postinjection Care

Apply pressure over injection sites. Have the patient ice the affected area for 20 minutes two to three times daily for the first 48–72 hours. Then begin local heat and gentle stretching exercises several days after the injection. Avoid vigorous exercise in the affected area for several days.

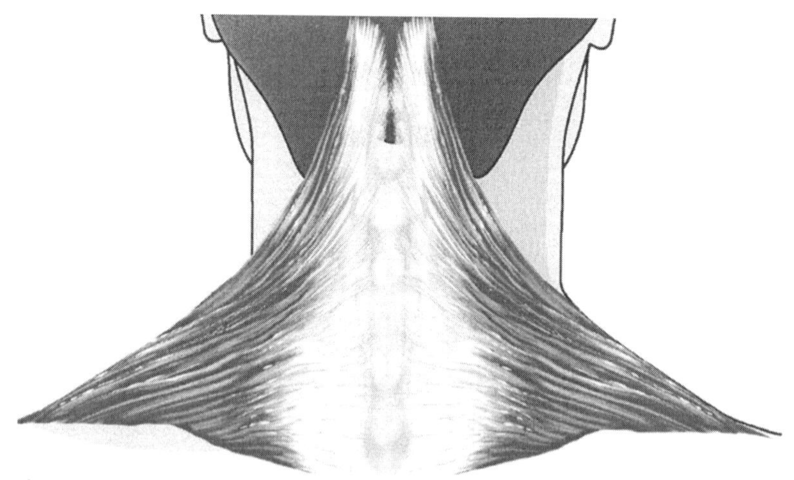

Fig 8–1 Botulinum toxin injection.

When to Perform Follow-Up Injections

Although there are no strict guidelines, a reasonable approach is to reinject every 3–4 months. Botulinum toxin is generally effective for approximately 12 weeks.

REFERENCES

Allam, N., Brasil-Neto, J. P., Brown, G., and Tomaz, C. (2005). Injections of botulinum toxin type A produce pain alleviation in intractable trigeminal neuralgia. *Clin. J. Pain* **21(2),** 182–184.

Charles, D. P. (2004). Botulinum neurotoxin serotype A: A clinical update on non-cosmetic uses. *Am. J. Health-Syst. Pharm.* **61(Suppl 6),** S11–S23.

Childers, M. K., and Simons, D. G. (2000). Botulinum toxin use in myofascial pain syndromes. *In* "Pain Procedures in Clinical Practice." (T. A. Lennard, Ed.). 2nd ed. pp. 191–192. Hanley and Belfus Publishers, Inc. Philadelphia, PA.

Ghazizadeh, S., and Nikzad, M. (2004). Botulinum toxin in the treatment of refractory vaginismus. *Obstet. Gynecol.* **104(5 Pt 1),** 913–914.

Naumann, M., and Jankovic, J. (2004). Safety of botulinum toxin type A: A systematic review and meta-analysis. *Curr. Med. Res. Opin.* **20(7),** 981–990.

Physician's Desk Reference. (2005) 59th ed. p. 563. Thomson PDR. Montvale, NJ.

Thomson, A. J., Jarvis, S. K., Lenart, M., Abbott, J. A., and Vancaillie, T. G. (2005). The use of botulinum toxin type A (Botox) as treatment for intractable chronic pelvic pain associated with spasm of the levator ani muscles. *Br. J. Obstet. Gynaecol.* **112(2),** 247–249.

9

Prolotherapy

Introduction

Prolotherapy, also known as regenerative injection therapy (RIT), is a form of treatment that involves the injection of ligaments or tendons with a proliferation agent such as dextrose. In theory, these ligaments and tendons that are injected are thought to demonstrate laxity or weakness that may be a primary pain generator. The proliferative solution is injected directly into the ligament or tendon at its bony attachment site. This solution is believed to stimulate fibroblast proliferation that restores normal connective tissue strength and length, which, in turn, reduces pain. This chapter will cover the historical aspects of prolotherapy, mechanism of action and clinical effectiveness, patient selection, and basic principles of the injection technique.

History

The principle of prolotherapy originated in the nonsurgical treatment of hemorrhoids, varicose veins, and hernias (Poritt, 1931). These conditions occur because of weakness in the connective tissue structures. Similarly, in ligaments and tendons, degeneration and laxity occur that sometimes results in chronic painful conditions. Early surgeons used a technique known as sclerotherapy on many of these conditions because the injection scarred or "sclerosed" the area. In the seventeenth century, Samuel Sharp taught medical students the technique of sclerotherapy on hydroceles. In 1938, Steindler and Luck provided strong evidence that ligaments and tendons were pain generators by the use of procaine injections (Steindler *et al.*, 1938). They were able to locate the noxious pain generators in the spine with the use of carefully injected procaine. In 1937, Schultz treated temporomandibular joint (TMJ) laxity with Synasal, a fatty acid solution. Injections were given into the TMJ joint capsule, and results were found to be effective and safe. This was probably the first true prolotherapy treatment recorded. G. S. Hackett is considered by most to be the father of prolotherapy. He advanced this form of treatment through research and teaching in the 1950s and coined the term "prolotherapy." He was one of the first to demonstrate ligament and tendon growth after proliferation treatments (Hackett, 1958; Hackett and Henderson, 1955). His student, Gustav Hemwall, MD, further advanced the technique of prolotherapy through his clinical treatments from 1955 until 1996 and has been called by many "the world's greatest prolotherapist."

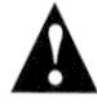

Mechanism of Action and Clinical Effectiveness

Prolotherapy injections usually contain various combinations of dextrose, phenol, saline, glycerine, or sodium morrhuate given in multiple sites. These injected sites are within the ligament or tendon proper where it attaches to bone. It is believed by prolotherapists that ligaments and tendons often heal poorly because of a limited blood supply. This incomplete healing may result in a lax or weak band of fibrous or connective tissue that becomes painful. It is postulated that once an injection is given, a localized inflammatory response occurs. This response stimulates a wound-healing cascade that includes an influx of fibroblasts. These fibroblastic cells deposit new collagen where the injection was given. As this new collagen matures, it shortens and strengthens the injected ligament or tendon. Microscopic studies have suggested the newly formed connective tissue has biomechanical properties similar to normal ligaments and tendons (Maynard *et al.*, 1985). Thus, the goal of prolotherapy is to restore normal tendon and ligament length and strength in the affected area. This restores skeletal support and reduces sources of myofascial trigger perpetuation (Hackett, 1958; Reeves, 2000).

The clinical effectiveness of prolotherapy has been well scrutinized. Its proponents believe it is a safe and effective method to treat chronic musculoskeletal pain, loss of motion, ligament laxity, and swelling. The literature is replete with research that describes its effectiveness on chronic low back pain, peripheral joint arthritic pain, anterior cruciate ligament (ACL) laxity, and temporomandibular joint (TMJ) pain (Hakala, 2005; Hooper and Ding, 2004; Linetsky *et al.,* 2000; 2001; Reeves, 2000; Topol *et al.*, 2005; Yelland *et al.*, 2004). Opponents argue there are limited high-quality data that support the use of prolotherapy in musculoskeletal conditions and that better research is needed (Dagenais *et al.*, 2005; Hooper and Ding, 2004; Kim *et al.*, 2004; Rabago *et al.*, 2005; Yelland, Del Mar *et al.*, 2004; Yelland, Glasziou *et al.*, 2004). Furthermore, it is thought that prolotherapy literature contains variable protocols, few participants, poorly defined objective measurements, and, often, anecdotal evidence.

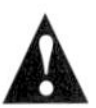

Patient Selection

In general, patients who experience symptoms consistent with joint laxity associated with pain may be candidates for proliferation therapy. These symptoms may include clicking, popping, or stiffness with limited range of joint motion. Many patients give histories of twisting or turning to pop their affected joint or spine for transient pain relief or to improve their range of motion. Some patients demonstrate balance or fatigue problems in certain joints, especially in the cervical spine. Many exhibit referred symptoms from tendons or ligaments that include pseudoradicular pain, tingling, or numbness. Before performing prolotherapy, basic diagnostic studies are necessary. These include plain x-rays and magnetic resonance (MR) imaging. These basic studies help to eliminate underlying fractures, congenital disorders, tumors, vascular anomalies, nerve root, disc, and meniscal injuries. In some cases, an MRI can define specific ligament or tendon disorders that may be a target for future proliferative treatments.

Prolotherapy is generally reserved for patients who have not improved with traditional forms of treatment such as rest, activity modification, medication, corticosteroid injections, physical therapy, and surgery. However, many practicing prolotherapists may begin injections as early as 8 weeks after an injury for strains and sprains, with the goal of reducing protracted treatment. Patients should be instructed to discontinue nonsteroidal anti-inflammatory drugs 3 days before treatment and 10 days afterward. Contraindications to prolotherapy are listed in Table 9–1.

Solutions Injected

The type of proliferant solution injected depends on the anatomical site that is being treated and the training and experience of the treating physician. Dextrose is the most

Table 9–1 Contraindications to Prolotherapy

1. Allergies to the proliferating agent
2. Acute joint dislocations
3. Septic joint
4. Posttraumatic hemarthrosis
5. Acute soft tissue injury
6. Acute gout or rheumatoid arthritis
7. Undiagnosed concomitant neurological disorder
8. Pregnancy (first trimester)

commonly used proliferant and is usually recommended for a patient's first treatment session. The Hackett method (Reeves *et al.*, 2000; 2003) uses predominantly dextrose solutions. Phenol-based solutions are commonly used to treat well-localized pain syndromes. The most widely used proliferant is dextrose based. See Table 9–2 for the various types of proliferant agents.

Injection Sites

The location of injection sites for prolotherapy is based on the knowledge of referral patterns from ligaments and tendons. These referral patterns have been well described (Reeves, 2000). For example, if a patient demonstrates isolated low back pain, the facet, lumbar intertransverse, iliolumbar, and sacroiliac ligaments will be injected. If buttock pain is also present in this example, the gluteal insertions, sacrospinous ligaments, articular hip ligaments, and external rotators of the hip will also be injected. If the pain extends into the thigh, the tendons of the distal knee adductors and hamstrings, knee capsule, and tendon of the vastus medialis may require injection. Figures 9–1 and 9–2 illustrate examples of the technique used for treating low back pain.

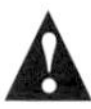

Injection Technique—Lumbar Spine Example

1. The patient is placed in the prone position with pillows and plinths for comfort.
2. The physician carefully palpates areas of tenderness in the lumbar spine.
3. Landmarks for injections are marked on the patient's low back. This includes the iliac crests, lumbar spinous processes, and PSIS. Avoid marking muscle trigger points.

Table 9–2 Proliferative Solutions

Dextrose-based solutions: Various dilutions with 1% lidocaine makes 10%, 12.5%, or 25% dextrose solutions.
Sodium morrhuate (usually 5%): A mixture of sodium salts of unsaturated and saturated fatty acids of cod liver oil and 2% benzyl alcohol (acts as an anesthetic and preservative).
Dextrose-phenol-glycerine (DPG or P2G) solutions; 25% dextrose/2.5% phenol/25% glycerine. This is usually diluted with a local anesthetic in a 1:1, 1:2, and 2:3 ratio.
Other solutions include 6% phenol in glycerine, tetracycline, chondroitin sulfate–glucosamine sulfate–dextrose solution.

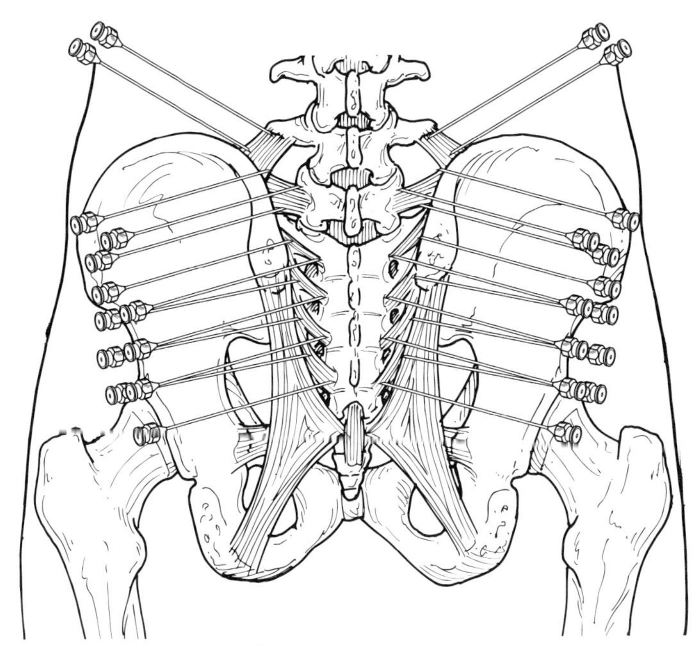

Fig 9–1 Prolotherapy injection sites.

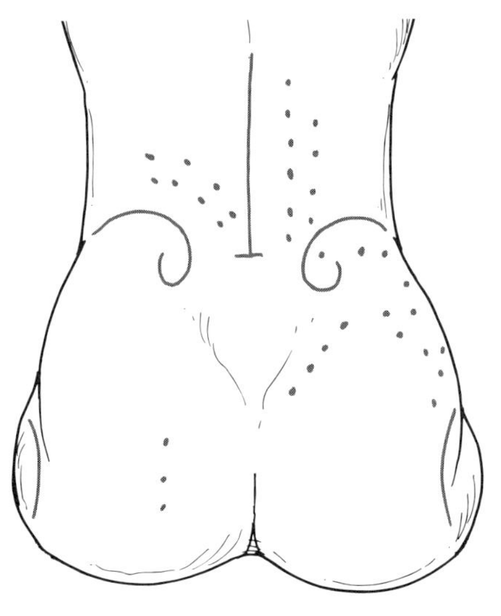

Fig 9–2 Prolotherapy injection sites noted on the skin surface.

4. Conscious sedation (optional) is given IV.
5. The patient's vital signs are closely monitored throughout the procedure.
6. The skin is cleaned with Betadine or Hibiclens.
7. Advance a 2- to 3-inch 25-gauge needle to bone adjacent to the desired ligament to be injected. Reposition the needle slightly into the ligament. In large patients, a 6-inch needle may be required.
8. Inject 1.5 mL of proliferative solution.
9. Withdraw the needle, and repeat the injection at multiple sites within the same ligament.
10. Repeat the same technique in other ligaments in the lumbar spine.
11. The patient is monitored after the procedure until stable and is discharged with a responsible driver.
12. The patient is encouraged to apply ice to the affected areas.

This same principle can be performed for most ligaments or tendons in other areas of the spine, peripheral joints, and soft tissue.

Conclusion

Prolotherapy has been used for decades for the treatment of painful musculoskeletal conditions. Its use requires proper patient selection and a good working knowledge of anatomy. One should always carefully examine and image the patient with chronic painful conditions before instituting proliferation therapy. Additional research is needed to further delineate proper patient selection and to verify outcomes after this form of treatment.

REFERENCES

Dagenais, S., Haldeman, S., and Wooley, J. R. (2005). Intraligamentous injection of sclerosing solutions (prolotherapy) for spinal pain: A critical review of the literature. *Spine J.* **5(3),** 310–328.

Hackett, G. (1958). Ligament and Tendon Relaxation (Skeletal Disability) Treated by Prolotherapy (Fibro-osseous Proliferation). 3rd ed. Charles C. Thomas, Springfield, IL.

Hackett, G., and Henderson, D. (1955). Joint stabilization: An experimental, histologic study with comments on the clinical application in ligament proliferation. *Am. J. Surg.* **89,** 968–973.

Hakala, R. V. (2005). Prolotherapy (proliferation therapy) in the treatment of TMD. *Cranio.* **23(4),** 283–288.

Hooper, R. A., and Ding, M. (2004). Retrospective case series on patients with chronic spinal pain treated with dextrose prolotherapy. *J. Altern. Complement Med.* **10(4),** 670–674.

Kim, S. R., Stitik, T. P., Foye, P. M., Greenwald, B. D., and Campagnolo, D. I. (2004). Critical review of prolotherapy for osteoarthritis, low back pain and other musculoskeletal conditions: A physiatric perspective. *Am. J. Phys. Med. Rehabil.* **83(5),** 379–389.

Linetsky, F., *et al.* (2000). Regenerative injection therapy: History of application in pain management, Part I 1930s–1950s. *Pain Clinic* **2(2),** 8–13.

Maynard, J., *et al.* (1985). Morphological and biochemical effects of sodium morrhuate on tendons. *J. Ortho. Res.* **3,** 234–248.

Poritt, A. (1931). The injection treatment of hydrocele, varicocele, bursae and nevi. *Proc. R. Soc. Med.* **24,** 81.

Rabago, D., Best, T. M., Beamsley, M., and Patterson, J. (2005). A systematic review of prolotherapy for chronic musculoskeletal pain. *Clin. J. Sport. Med.* **15(5),** E376.

Reeves, K. D. (2000). Prolotherapy: Basic science, clinical studies, and technique. *In* Pain Procedures in Clinical Practice. 2nd ed. (T. A. Lennard, Ed.), pp. 172–190. Hanley and Belfus, London.

Reeves, K. D., and Hassanein, K. (2000). Randomized prospective double-blind placebo-controlled study of dextrose prolotherapy for knee osteoarthritis with or without ACL laxity. *Altern. Ther. Health Med.* **6(2),** 68–74, 77–80.

Reeves, K. D., and Hassanein, K. (2000). Randomized, prospective, placebo-controlled double-blind study of dextrose prolotherapy for osteoarthritic thumb and finger joints: Evidence of clinical efficacy. *J. Altern. Complement Med.* **6(4),** 311–320.

Reeves, K. D., and Hassanein, K. (2003). Long-term effects of dextrose prolotherapy for anterior cruciate ligament laxity. *Altern. Ther. Health Med.* **9(3),** 58–62.

Steindler, A., *et al.* (1938). Differential diagnosis of pain low in the back; allocation of the source of pain by the procaine hydrochloride method. *JAMA* **110,** 106–113.

Topol, G. A., Reeves, K. D., and Hassanein, K. M. (2005). Efficacy of dextrose prolotherapy in elite male kicking-sport athletes with chronic groin pain. *Arch. Phys. Med. Rehabil.* **86(4),** 697–702.

Yelland, M. J., Del Mar, C., Pirozzo, S., and Schoene, M. L. (2004). Prolotherapy injections for chronic low back pain: A systematic review. *Spine* **29(19),** 2126–2133.

Yelland, M. J., Glasziou, P. P., Bogduk, N., Schluter, P. J., and McKernon, M. (2004). Prolotherapy injections, saline injections, and exercises for chronic low-back pain: A randomized trial. *Spine* **29(1),** 9–16; discussion 16.

10

Acupuncture

Acupuncture is one of the best examples of nontraditional treatment that after much research is now considered a conventional therapy for a number of different conditions and symptoms including musculoskeletal pain. There are several schools of thought—the most popular ones stemming from Chinese, Japanese, and French traditions. In this chapter, we will discuss acupuncture that originates from traditional Chinese medicine (TCM).

Acupuncture is part of TCM that dates back several thousand years. TCM follows three main principles that include yin and yang, chi, or qi, and the five element theory (Shankar and Liao, 2004). Yin and yang refer to the interaction between opposing forces in the body. These terms are used to describe how things react with respect to each other. Neither yin nor yang is better than the other—the importance is balance. Yin delineates such things as femininity, dark, and cold. Yang is composed of masculinity, light, and warm. In the earl days of TCM, it was believed that everything had a yin and a yang component. Things could only be described when both the yin and the yang were understood. For example, people understood what warm was when they had experienced cold. Ultimately, the goal with TCM, which includes acupuncture and herbal medicine, is to restore the balance between yin and yang.

Another concept that is a mainstay of TCM is chi, which refers to the vital energy that flows in the body and is essential for life. The general theory is that there are patterns of energy flow (qi) within the body that are important to maintain good health. Ancient theory dictates that disruptions in these patterns leads to illness.

The final component of TCM is the five element theory that is based on five essential elements: wood, fire, earth, metal, and water. This is a fairly complicated concept; however, these five elements basically correlate to five human organs—lungs, heart, kidneys, spleen, and liver.

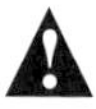

Mechanism of Action

Acupuncture involves the systematic insertion of very fine needles (usually between 32 and 36 gauge) into specific, predetermined points in the body. These points are called acupuncture points or acu points and correspond to meridians throughout the body (Figures 10–1 through 10–5). There are more than 350 acupuncture points that lie along the meridians. It is believed that chi (or the body's vital energy) flows through these meridians. Where the needles are placed depends on a number of factors, including whether the objective is to consolidate or disperse the chi.

Acupuncture has been studied fairly extensively, and over the last several decades, the scientific evidence has substantiated that acupuncture stimulation (with needles alone) and electroacupuncture stimulation (with needles and an electrical stimulator)

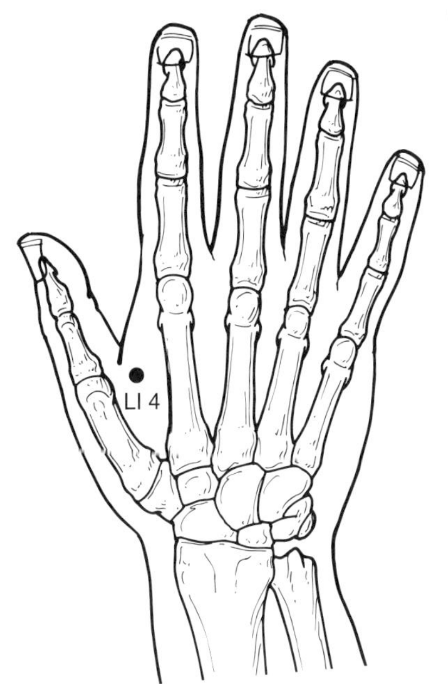

Fig 10–1 Acupuncture points: large intestine 4 (LI4).

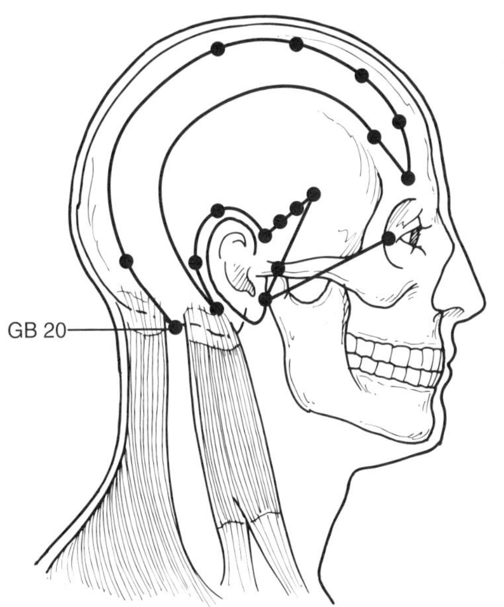

Fig 10–2 Acupuncture points: gallbladder 20 (GB20).

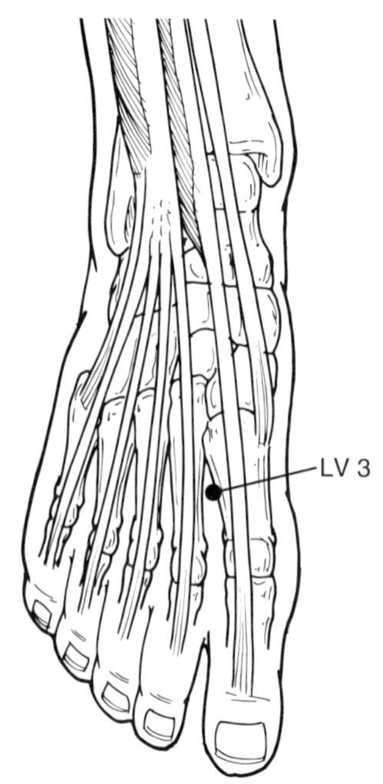

Fig 10–3 Acupuncture points: liver 3 (LV3).

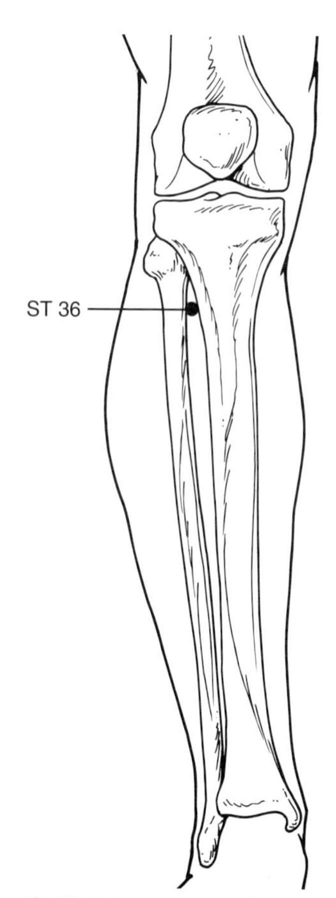

Fig 10–4 Acupuncture points: stomach 36 (ST36).

have physiological effects that influence the neurohormonal systems that modulate pain. We know from this research that acupuncture releases endorphins and enkephalins in the central nervous system (CNS) and that these neuropeptides play a role in analgesia.

The many potential benefits of acupuncture include pain relief and perhaps improved healing from an acute or chronic injury (Table 10–1). For example,

> At the Winter Olympics in Japan in 1998, international exposure came when the acupuncturists in Nagano offered free treatments to Olympic athletes and officials, emphasizing that it is a drug-free way to treat injuries. Even more stunning was the near miraculous recovery in response to acupuncture by the Austrian, Hermann Maier. Maier won gold medals in the giant slalom super G 3 days after a dramatic fall and injury that occurred during the downhill competition. Maier mentioned to the press that the use of acupuncture to treat his shoulder and knee injuries after the fall helped him to recover (Silver and Audette, 2003).

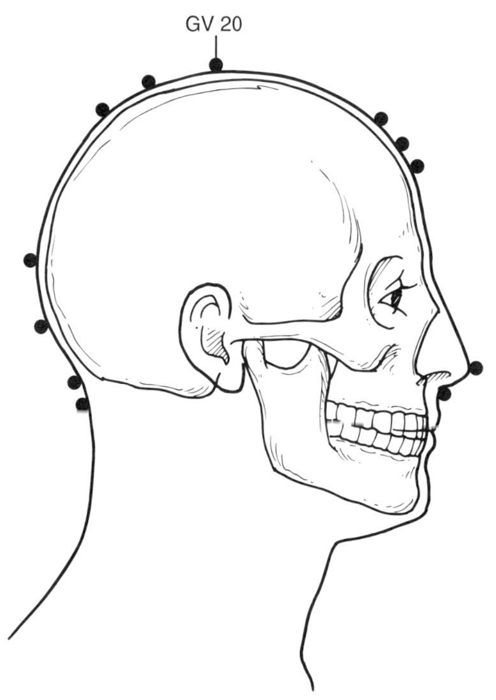

Fig 10–5 Acupuncture points: governor vessel 20 (GV20).

Table 10–1 Evidence-Based Indications for Acupuncture[1]

Considered effective	Probably effective	Promising early research but unclear whether effective	Research is inconclusive	Probably not effective
Postoperative dental pain	Low back pain	Fibromyalgia	Chronic pain	Smoking cessation
Postoperative nausea and vomiting	Migraine	Osteoarthritis	Neck pain	Tinnitus
Chemotherapy-related nausea and vomiting	Temporomandibular disorders	Tennis elbow	Asthma	Weight loss
			Drug addiction	

[1]From Birch, S., Hesselink, J. K., Jonkman, F., Hekker, T., and Bos, A. (2004). Clinical research on acupuncture: Part 1. What have reviews of the efficacy and safety of acupuncture told us so far? *J. Altern. Complementary Med.* **10(3),** 468–480.

Ironically it was President Nixon's visit to China in 1972 that led to an explosion of American interest in this and other Eastern therapies. Twenty-five years after Nixon's visit, the National Institutes of Health (NIH) convened a panel of experts including physicians, scientists, and alternative medicine practitioners to review the research on acupuncture. In 1997, adhering to the panel's recommendations, NIH released a "consensus statement" with the following conclusion:

"...promising results have emerged, for example, efficacy of acupuncture in adult post-operative and chemotherapy nausea and vomiting and in postoperative dental pain. There are other situations such as addiction, stroke rehabilitation, headache, menstrual cramps, tennis elbow, fibromyalgia, myofascial pain, osteoarthritis, low back pain, carpal tunnel syndrome, and asthma for which acupuncture may be useful as an adjunct treatment or an acceptable alternative or be included in a comprehensive management program. Further research is likely to uncover additional areas where acupuncture interventions will be useful.

Findings from basic research have begun to elucidate the mechanisms of action of acupuncture, including the release of opioids and other peptides in the central nervous system and the periphery and changes in neuroendocrine function. Although much needs to be accomplished, the emergence of plausible mechanisms for the therapeutic effects of acupuncture is encouraging.

The introduction of acupuncture into the choice of treatment modalities readily available to the public is in its early stages. Issues of training, licensure, and reimbursement remain to be clarified. There is sufficient evidence, however, of its potential value to conventional medicine to encourage further studies.

There is sufficient evidence of acupuncture's value to expand its use into conventional medicine and to encourage further studies of its physiology and clinical value (NIH Consensus Statement, 1997).

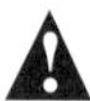

Potential Risks

Acupuncture is believed to be quite safe with few inherent risks when performed with sterile needles by someone who is skilled. There are very rare adverse events described in the literature, including cardiac tamponade, pneumothorax, and transmission of diseases such as hepatitis (Birch *et al.*, 2004). Systemic anticoagulation is not a strict contraindication, but one should be careful in a patient with an elevated INR. Patients with severe hemophilia or other potentially uncontrolled bleeding disorders should not undergo acupuncture. This modality should be used in caution in pregnant women to avoid "forbidden" points that may stimulate uterine contractility.

Electroacupuncture should not be used in patients with a history of seizures or epilepsy or in people with heart disease who have pacemakers. It should also not be performed on a patient's head, throat, or directly over the heart. Another precaution that is somewhat disputed is that when needles are being connected to an electric current, the current should not travel across the midline of the body (an imaginary line running from the bridge of the nose to the umbilicus). There have never been any studies to show that electric current that crosses the midline poses a health risk to the patient; however, some acupuncturists believe it is important to adhere to this precaution.

Minor adverse events are not unusual, and these include transitory pain from the needle, local bleeding and/or bruising, and vasovagal responses such as light-headedness and fainting.

Acupuncture is widely accepted as a form of complimentary/alternative medicine (CAM) that works for a variety of medical conditions. Many insurers still do not cover this modality, however. It is often reimbursed by Workers' Compensation, and some HMO plans pay for it as well. Medicare and Medicaid do not currently cover this form of treatment. Physicians who are trained in acupuncture may bill the initial evaluation as a consultation visit or standard E & M code. A reasonable trial of acupuncture is a series of 4–10 visits.

Readers who are interested in further training in this technique may take one of several courses offered in affiliation with accredited medical schools. Many of the procedures in this book can be performed by physicians without a lot of additional training; however, acupuncture is not one of these. To be a skilled acupuncturist, one must devote considerable time to understanding the practice and learning the technique. This chapter is an introduction to acupuncture, and interested readers should pursue further guidance and training elsewhere.

REFERENCES

Birch, S., Hesselink, J. K., Jonkman, F., Hekker, T., and Bos, A. (2004). Clinical research on acupuncture: Part 1. What have reviews of the efficacy and safety of acupuncture told us so far? *J. Altern. Complementary Med.* **10(3),** 474.

NIH Consensus Statement. (1997). Acupuncture. **15(5),** 1–34.

Shankar, K., and Liao, L. P. (2004). Traditional systems of medicine. *Phys. Med. Rehabil. Clin. North Am.* **15,** 725–747.

Silver, J. K., and Audette, J. (2003). Pharmacological agents and acupuncture in rehabilitation. *In* Rehabilitation of Sports Injuries: Scientific Basis. (W. R. Frontera, Ed.). p. 198. Blackwell Publishing. Malden, MA.

11

Sympathetic Injections

Sympathetic injections are useful procedures in patients who have suspected sympathetic mediated pain. Hyperactivity of the sympathetic nervous system may be responsible for many disorders and presents with varying symptoms. These symptoms and pain problems may include migraine or cluster headaches; facial neuralgias; and intractable ocular, pelvic, retroperitoneal, or perineal pain. Sympathetic blocks can be used to mitigate pain from these symptoms and to treat pain from cancer, acute pancreatitis, and complex regional pain syndrome (CRPS), type I or II. CRPS was formerly referred to as reflex sympathetic dystrophy. Current nomenclature is CRPS Type I, which follows trauma without a specific nerve injury, and CRPS Type II, which develops after injury to a nerve.

This chapter will focus on the injection treatment of CRPS by reviewing pertinent sympathetic injection anatomy, discussing diagnostic criteria of complex regional pain syndrome, and outlining details of cervical stellate ganglion and lumbar sympathetic blocks. Injection techniques for collateral ganglia, splanchnic nerves, sphenopalatine and gasserian ganglion, superior hypogastric plexus, ganglion impar, and celiac plexus blocks are beyond the scope of this chapter.

Injection Anatomy of the Sympathetic System

The paired sympathetic trunk or chain extends along the length of the vertebral column with each side consisting of a series of 22 paravertebral sympathetic ganglia. Preganglionic neurons that arise from the central nervous system synapse in these paravertebral ganglia with their postganglionic neurons ultimately extend to the effector organ (e.g., smooth muscle, skin, glands, cardiac). Other preganglionic sympathetic neurons bypass these paravertebral ganglia and synapse near vessels in collateral ganglia. Collateral ganglia are typically named after nearby blood vessels. Groups of these collateral ganglia are referred to as a plexus, and their postganglionic neurons are often collectively called splanchnic nerves.

The sympathetic innervation to the upper extremities and head originates from the fifth through seventh thoracic segments of the spinal cord. Their preganglionic fibers synapse in the cervical sympathetic chain in the superior, middle, or inferior ganglia. These upper two ganglia lie just anterior to the longus colli and capitis muscles, posterior to the carotid sheath, and medial to the vertebral artery. The postganglionic fibers from the superior cervical ganglion supply the C1–4 nerve roots and the cardiac plexus. Those fibers from the middle cervical ganglion supply the C5 and C6 nerve roots along with the cardiac plexus and thyroid gland. The inferior cervical ganglion is often fused with the first thoracic ganglia and forms the stellate ganglion. Postganglionic fibers from this ganglion supply the C7, C8, and T1 nerve roots and the vertebral plexus.

The sympathetic innervation to the lower extremities originates from the lower thoracic and upper lumbar spinal cord segments. Their preganglionic fibers synapse in the lumbar sympathetic chain ganglia. Postganglionic fibers supply the lumbar nerve roots. Usually a lumbar sympathetic block at the L1–L3 levels will affect the lower extremities.

The proximity of the sympathetic chain to the vertebral column in both the cervical and lumbar spine makes it easily accessible for an injection. Fluoroscopy and contrast agents are routinely used to improve the accuracy and safety of these injections. Meticulous attention to detail and a solid knowledge of the regional anatomy is necessary for a successful block.

Complex Regional Pain Syndrome

Complex regional pain syndrome is a chronic painful condition that normally affects an arm or leg after a soft tissue, nerve, or bone injury (Allen *et al.*, 1999; Purdy and Miller, 1992; Veldman *et al.*, 1993). The pathophysiology of this disorder is poorly understood but, in general, is believed to occur as a result of a hyperactive sympathetic nervous system. This condition was first described by Mitchell in his article published in 1864 entitled "Gunshot Wounds and Other Injuries of Nerves" (Mitchell *et al.*, 1864). Historically, there have been a number of names for CRPS, including Sudeck's atrophy, sympathalgia, minor causalgia, shoulder hand syndrome, posttraumatic spreading neuralgia, and reflex sympathetic dystrophy (RSD). In 1994, the International Association for the Study of Pain adopted uniform nomenclature and now recommends the term complex regional pain syndrome (CRPS) types I and II in place of reflex sympathetic dystrophy (RSD) and causalgia (Racz *et al.*, 1996). It was generally agreed that the term CRPS would be more representative of the broad spectrum of clinical symptoms seen in this condition.

The diagnosis of CRPS I and II is based on clinical findings. No single diagnostic study exists to confirm this disorder. The diagnostic criteria for CRPS type I (RSD) and II (causalgia) can be found in Tables 11–1 and 11–2. Type I occurs when a nerve injury cannot be immediately identified. By contrast, type II exists when a specific nerve has been injured. The symptoms from CRPS I and II include various combinations of swelling, sweating, skin mottling, hair and nail changes, sensory changes, weakness, and burning pain out of proportion to what one would expect. In most cases, these symptoms are isolated to one extremity. In type II, there may be concomitant findings consistent with a nerve injury such as focal numbness, weakness, or atrophy in the distribution of the injured nerve. Because CRPS advances, muscles atrophy, joints stiffen, tendons contract, swelling worsens, and regional bones may develop general demineralization.

Table 11–1 Diagnostic Criteria for Complex Regional Pain Syndrome Type I

1. The presence of prior immobilization or a noxious event.
2. Pain, allodynia, or hyperalgesia disproportionate to the expected injury.
3. Abnormal regional sudomotor activity or edema and changes in skin blood flow such as skin temperature changes (>1.1° C difference from the contralateral body part) and skin color changes.
4. Other etiologies of the symptoms have been excluded.

Table 11–2 Diagnostic Criteria for Complex Regional Pain Syndrome Type II

1. The presence of a nerve injury with pain, allodynia, or hyperalgesia. This does not have to be limited to the distribution of the injured nerve.

1. Abnormal regional sudomotor activity or edema and changes in skin blood flow such as skin temperature changes (>1.1° C difference from the contralateral body part) and skin color changes.
2. Other etiologies of the symptoms have been excluded.

Patient Selection for Sympathetic Injections

Patients with CRPS I or II may benefit from either single or multiple sympathetic anesthetic blocks. In general, it has been accepted that the injections should be performed as early as possible within the treatment algorithm of this disorder. A single sympathetic anesthetic injection can confirm one's clinical suspicion of the working diagnosis. For example, if a patient is seen with unilateral upper extremity burning pain associated with mild swelling, and temperature changes and other diagnostic imaging and electrical studies have been normal, an anesthetic diagnostic cervical sympathetic block may be indicated. The patient's response to the injection immediately after the procedure can be monitored to determine whether their preinjection symptoms have changed or subsided. If the patient's symptoms are temporarily relieved and this relief can be reproduced with future blocks and their symptoms correspond to the criteria discussed in Tables 11–1 or 11–2, the diagnosis of complex regional pain syndrome may be confirmed. Once the diagnosis of CRPS has been confirmed, additional sympathetic injections can be performed to reduce symptoms and to allow range of motion and exercises to the affected limb. Unfortunately, no clear guidelines exist on the number or frequency of these injections. In fact, the literature is quite divisive on this issue, and even their efficacy has come into question (Baron *et al.*, 2003; Hogan and Hurwitz, 2002; Hord and Oaklander, 2003; Quisel *et al.*, 2005).

Sympathetic injections are relatively safe when good technique is followed and patients are appropriately selected. These injections are contraindicated in medically unstable patients, those on blood thinners, or those who have active systemic infections. Once an injection has started, IV access should be available, and the patient's blood pressure, pulse oximetry, EKG, and heart rate should be monitored. After the injection, careful monitoring of the patient is critical, and any changes in the preinjection symptoms are recorded. The patient should also undergo range of motion exercises to the affected limb during the postinjection period. Many physicians have their patient scheduled for postinjection physical therapy during this period.

Cervical Stellate Ganglion Blocks CPT Code 64510 (Stellate Ganglion or Cervical Sympathetic)

Bilateral blockade is not recommended because of the risk of hypoventilation from a phrenic nerve block or aspiration from a recurrent laryngeal nerve block (Figures 11–1 and 11–2).

1. The patient is placed in the supine position with the jaw relaxed and the neck slightly extended.
2. By use of fluoroscopy, the C6 and C7 vertebral bodies are marked.

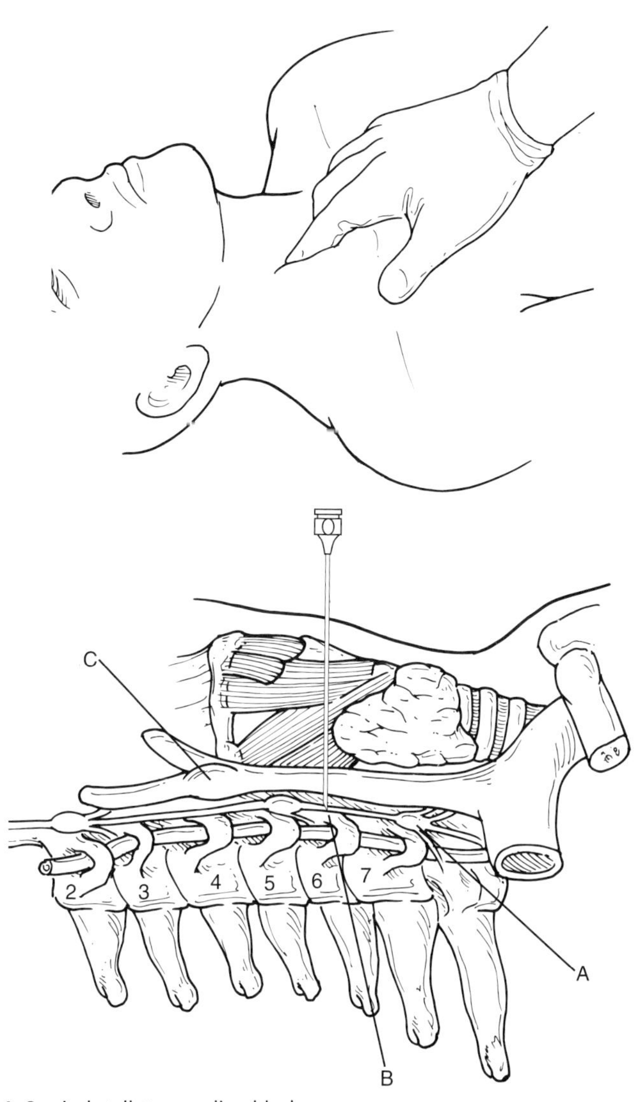

Fig 11–1 Cervical stellate ganglion block.

3. Betadine or Hibiclens is used to scrub the skin, and sterile drapes are applied to the field.
4. The carotid sheath is carefully retracted laterally and the larynx medially to allow the physician's fingertip to palpate for the anterior body of C7 or the bony protuberance at the base of the C6 transverse process.
5. Three to five cubic centimeters of 1% lidocaine is used to anesthetize the skin and subcutaneous tissue.
6. Under fluoroscopy, a 1½- or 3½-inch 22- or 25-gauge spinal needle is inserted until contact is made with the C6 or C7 anterior vertebral body and then withdrawn approximately 1 cm.

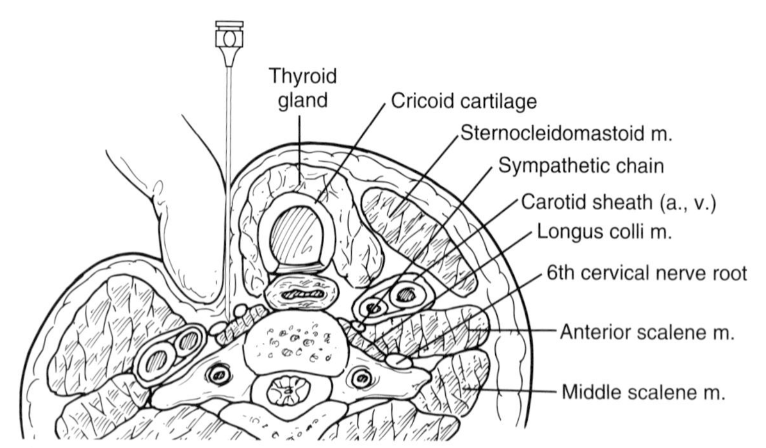

Fig 11–2 Cross-sectional anatomy of the neck demonstrating needle placement during a cervical sympathetic ganglion block.

7. Inject 3–5 cc of contrast. The column of contrast should extend in both a cephalad and caudal direction of the spine. Careful evaluation of the contrast pattern should be noted and should not be seen to flow into the neuroforamen or any vascular structure.
8. Inject a test dose of 0.2–0.5 cc of anesthetic solution and monitor the patient closely for signs of intravascular injection.
9. A total of 6–10 cc of 0.25% or 0.5% bupivacaine can be injected.
10. A successful block is demonstrated by the patient developing a Horner's syndrome (ipsilateral ptosis, partial ptosis of the upper eyelid), miosis (ipsilateral pupillary constriction), and anhydrosis (lack of facial sweating on the ipsilateral side) and a 2° C temperature increase in the ipsilateral upper extremity.

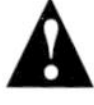

Lumbar Sympathetic Blocks CPT Code 64520 Lumbar or Thoracic (Paravertebral Sympathetics)

Bilateral blockade is not recommended because of the potential risk of hypotension (Figure 11–3).

1. The patient is placed in a prone position under fluoroscopy.
2. A skin mark is made at the location where the fluoroscopic beam is rotated until the tip of the L2 transverse process is superimposed directly over the body of the L2 vertebrae.
3. Betadine or Hibiclens is used to scrub the skin, and sterile drapes are applied to the field.
4. The skin, subcutaneous tissue, and muscle are anesthetized with 3–5 cc of 1% lidocaine.
5. A 3½- or 6-inch 22- or 25-gauge spinal needle is inserted under fluoroscopic guidance directly toward and beyond the tip of the L2 transverse process until it contacts the inferior anterolateral L2 vertebral body. On a sagittal view, the needle tip should be within the longitudinal interpedicular line.
6. Five to six cubic centimeters of contrast are injected and should be observed to extend up and down the thoracolumbar spine.

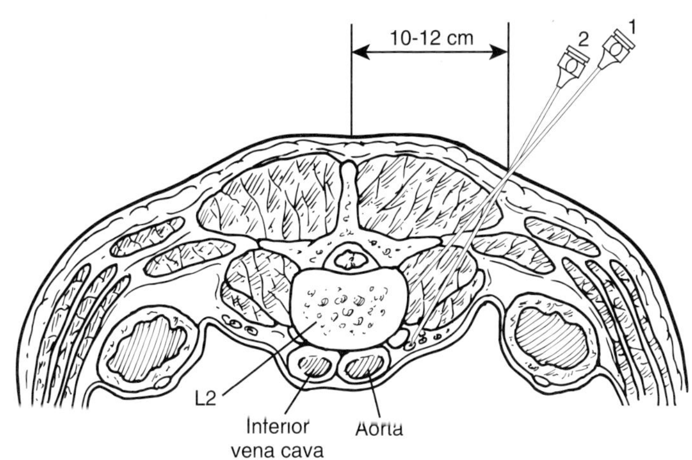

Fig 11–3 Lumbar sympathetic block.

7. Inject 10–15 cc of 0.25% or 0.5% of bupivacaine.
8. A successful block is indicated by a rise in lower extremity skin temperature of 3° C.

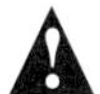

Conclusions

Sympathetic injections are a useful procedure for sympathetic mediated pain problems. These procedures require specialized training and a solid knowledge of regional anatomy and the ability to care for complications. Although their effectiveness has been questioned, these procedures are commonly used for diagnostic purposes and can often reduce a patient's pain complaints.

REFERENCES

Allen, G., *et al.* (1999). Epidemiological review of 134 patients with complex regional pain syndromes assessed in a chronic pain clinic. *Pain* **80,** 539–544.

Baron, R., Binder, A., Ulrich, W., and Maier, C. (2003). Complex regional pain syndrome. Sympathetic reflex dystrophy and causalgia. *Schmerz* **17(3),** 213–226.

Hogan, C. J., and Hurwitz, S. R. (2002). Treatment of complex regional pain syndrome of the lower extremity. *J. Am. Acad. Orthop. Surg.* **10(4),** 281–289.

Hord, E. D., and Oaklander, A. L. (2003). Complex regional pain syndrome: A review of evidence-supported treatment options. *Curr. Pain Headache Rep.* **7(3),** 188–196.

Mitchell, S. W., Morehouse, G. R., and Keen, W. W. (1864). Gunshot Wounds and Injuries of Nerves. J. B. Lippincott, New York.

Purdy, C. A., and Miller, S. J. (1992). Reflex sympathetic dystrophy syndrome. *In* Comprehensive Textbook of Foot Surgery. 2nd ed. pp. 1124–1134. Williams and Wilkins, London.

Quisel, A., Gill, J. M., and Witherell, P. (2005). Complex regional pain syndrome: Which treatments show promise? *J. Fam. Pract.* **54(7),** 599–603.

Racz, G. B., Heavener, J. E., and Noe, C. E. (1996). Definitions, classifications and taxonomy: An overview. *Phys. Med. Rehabil. State Art Rev.* **10,** 195–206.

Veldman, P. J. M., *et al.* (1993). Signs and symptoms of reflex sympathetic dystrophy: Prospective study of 829 patients. *Lancet* **342,** 1012–1016.

12

Spinal Injections

Spinal injections play an integral part in the diagnosis and treatment of spinal pain and dysfunction. These procedures can be useful during the diagnostic phase of treatment by precisely localizing the pain generator within the spinal compartment. They can also be helpful in determining whether suspicious segmental abnormalities seen on imaging studies are, in fact, a source of pain. Thus, they can be both diagnostic and therapeutic. In addition, some sources suggest these procedures can assist in predicting future surgical outcomes (Derby *et al.*, 1992). In the treatment of the painful spine, injections have the potential to reduce or eliminate the painful stimulus, thereby advancing the patient's overall functional status. In many of these cases, simply experiencing a reduction in their pain, either temporary or permanent, can be just enough to allow both their functional and psychological status to improve. The importance of a concomitant spinal rehabilitation program addressing spinal conditioning, weight management, flexibility, smoking cessation, and other necessary behavior and lifestyle changes clearly improves the patient's recovery and outcome (Botwin *et al.*, 2002; Krames, 1999; Tong *et al.*, 2004). A concomitant spinal rehabilitation program complements the spinal injection.

Patient Selection

Recognizing which patients may benefit from spinal injections is a key component to success. For most patients, injections should be performed within the framework of broader rehabilitation goals. For example, spinal exercises and oral medications may be appropriate for many patients and often will obviate the need for injection. It is important to note that spinal injections are usually not a first-line treatment option, and more conservative measures should be tried before considering injections.

When an injection is contemplated, x-rays and other imaging studies should be performed to eliminate the possibility of the unexpected fracture, infection, or tumor and to help localize the source of the pain. Advanced imaging studies such as MRI can be used, along with the physical examination, to determine the specific type and location of the injection to be done. Patients who experience spine pain refractory to routine conservative treatment such as modality and exercise-based physical therapy and soft tissue and manual forms of treatment including some forms of manipulative therapy, oral medications, and activity modification may be candidates for injections. Although no strict criteria exist on the timing of the initial injection, most physicians will wait a minimum of 4–8 weeks from the onset of the pain. In cases of severe spinal or radicular symptoms, it may be prudent to proceed sooner to accomplish functional goals.

Before an injection, it is important to obtain a thorough medical history. One should inquire about drug allergies, current medications, and medical conditions. Spinal injections should not be performed on patients taking blood thinners such as coumarin, aspirin, or other antiplatelet drugs or on women who may be pregnant. Injections are also contraindicated in patients who have systemic infections or an immunosuppressed condition. Patients with diabetes should be cautioned about a transient elevation of their blood glucose when corticosteroids are used.

The number of injections that a patient may reasonably undergo has not been determined. At present, it is generally acceptable, and often routine, to perform up to three epidural injections on patients, but limited data support these numbers. In fact, it seems that if the initial injection is not successful, a second injection is unlikely to be beneficial (Kaplan and Derby, 1998).

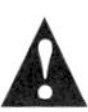

Who Is Qualified to Perform Spinal Injections?

Specialized training and a keen interest are required to become proficient in spinal injections. The physician who performs these injections should be confident in radiographic, surface, and spinal anatomy; well versed in the treatment of spinal disorders; educated on proper patient selection; and able to recognize and treat any complications that may arise from the procedure. A multitude of medical and surgical specialists are reported in the International Spinal Injection Society (ISIS) as currently performing spinal injections and include physiatrists, anesthesiologists, orthopedic and neurological surgeons, neurologists, radiologists, rheumatologists, internists, and general practitioners. Many physicians establish and rekindle their procedural skills through courses taught by ISIS and other organizations. Clearly, this is helpful, but it cannot replace supervised and proctored learning. Residency programs and pain management fellowships are available that train physicians in these spinal injection skills.

What Equipment Is Necessary?

The basic setup for a spinal procedure room differs very little from other medical or surgical procedure rooms. One exception may be the necessity of C-arm fluoroscopy and its accompanying adjustable height table. It is now standard practice to perform spinal injections with the use of fluoroscopy. Other suggested equipment is listed in Table 12–1.

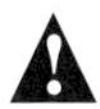

Potential Complications

Before performing a spinal injection, the physician should carefully review with the patient potential side effects of the procedure. These side effects may be from the procedure itself or the medications injected. A physician who chooses to perform spinal injections should be keenly aware of these potential pitfalls and be prepared to manage them aggressively.

Frequent side effects include:

1. Soreness at the injection site.
2. Vasovagal response during the procedure.
3. Corticosteroid reactions—facial flushing, tachycardia, chest pain, extremity swelling, headaches, feeling of malaise, fever, mood swings, elevated glucose.
4. Contrast agent reaction—headaches.
5. Bleeding.
6. Dural puncture headache.

Table 12–1 Procedure Room Equipment

1. C-arm fluoroscopy
2. Cardioversion equipment
3. Oxygen
4. Intubation supplies
5. IV trays
6. Medications for resuscitation
7. Stretcher and/or wheelchair
8. Surgical trays that include s terile 4 × 4s, 5-cc plastic syringes, tubing, drapes
9. Betadine or Hibiclens
10. Needles including for skin (27 gauge), drawing medications (18 gauge)
11. Spinal needles—3½-inch 25-gauge, 3½-inch 22-gauge, 18- or 20-gauge Tuohy
12. Glass syringes
13. Lidocaine 0.5%, 1%, 2%
14. Marcaine 0.5%
15. Contrast agents
16. Corticosteroids - Depo-Medrol
17. Sterile water
18. Band-Aids, tape
The procedure room should also be staffed with properly trained personnel who understand spinal injections, C-arm fluoroscopy operations, and can recognize and treat emerging complications or problems when they occur.

Less common side effects include:

1. Allergic reactions.
2. Local or systemic infection; epidural abscess.
3. Epidural hematoma.
4. Anesthetic toxicity.

Central nervous system effects—anxiety, circumoral or tongue numbness, metallic taste in mouth, nausea, dizziness, drowsiness, tremors or twitching, seizures, coma, respiratory arrest.

Cardiovascular effects—peripheral vasodilation, myocardial depression, angina, bradycardia, arrhythmias, cardiac arrest.

5. Traumatic neurovascular injury.

Injections directed toward the cervical spine deserve special precautions given the proximity to the vertebral or radicular artery. Spinal cord infarction has been reported from the development of a thrombosis of a reinforcing artery or embolization of the anterior spinal artery from corticosteroid particulate material (Brouwers *et al.*, 1991). The physician must absolutely understand the severity of causing a high spinal block when anesthetics are inadvertently injected into the subarachnoid space. In addition, paraplegia has been reported after lumbar transforaminal epidurals as a result of an anatomical variant involving a dominant left-sided radiculomedullary artery at the L1, L2, and L3 levels (Houton and Errico, 2002). One potential, and sometimes unavoidable, complication is a dural puncture headache. This occurs when the spinal needle is advanced beyond the epidural space and through the dural sac. As a result, cerebrospinal fluid may transiently leak from the puncture site causing severe headaches. Treatment of this complication is bed rest, hydration, caffeine, and, when protracted or severe, an epidural blood patch can be performed.

Spinal Injection Anatomy

The spine can be divided into the anterior, neuroaxial, and posterior compartments. The anterior compartment consists of the intervertebral disc and the vertebral body. The neuroaxial compartment includes the structures within the ligamentous and bony boundaries of the spinal canal, which include the epidural space, ligamentum flavum, posterior longitudinal ligament, and the neural structures. The posterior compartment includes the zygapophyseal or z-joints (facet joints). Subtle anatomical changes within each compartment can be observed when one compares the cervical, thoracic, lumbar, and sacral regions of the spine.

The types of spinal injections can be broadly categorized on the basis of these three spinal compartments. Injections into the *anterior compartment* would include discograms, nucleoplasty, percutaneous discectomy, intradiscal electrotherapy (IDET), kyphoplasty, and vertebroplasty. In each of these procedures, the target location for the needle or probe is within either the intervertebral disc or the vertebral body. Specific details of these procedures are beyond the scope of this chapter. Injections into the *neuroaxial compartment* consist primarily of epidurals. Epidural injections can be differentiated on the basis of their anatomical entry point and include midline, paramedian, transforaminal, and caudle approaches. The first three approaches can be performed at most spinal levels, with a few exceptions in the upper cervical spine. The caudal approach is limited to the hiatus between the sacral cornu. Injections into the *posterior compartment* consist of intra-articular z-joint, medial branch nerve blocks, sacroiliac joint, and radiofrequency neurotomies. Although the atlantooccipital and the lateral atlantoaxial joints in the upper cervical spine are not technically z-joints because of their anterior location, injections into these structures can be included within the posterior compartment.

Loss of Resistance Technique (Figure 12–1)

For Midline or Paramedian Epidural Injections

1. Use a small-volume glass syringe, 2–5 cc.
2. Lubricate the inner plunger of the syringe with a few drops of lidocaine.
3. Attach the syringe to a Tuohy needle.
4. Fully withdraw the plunger and advance the needle tip through the skin and into the interspinous ligament (midline) or ligamentum flavum (paramedian) while light downward pressure is applied against the tip of the plunger.
5. There should be moderate resistance to efforts made to advance the plunger.
6. Slowly and carefully advance the needle tip through the ligamentum flavum while maintaining pressure on the plunger.
7. When the needle tip enters the epidural space, a sudden loss of resistance is felt on the end of the plunger.

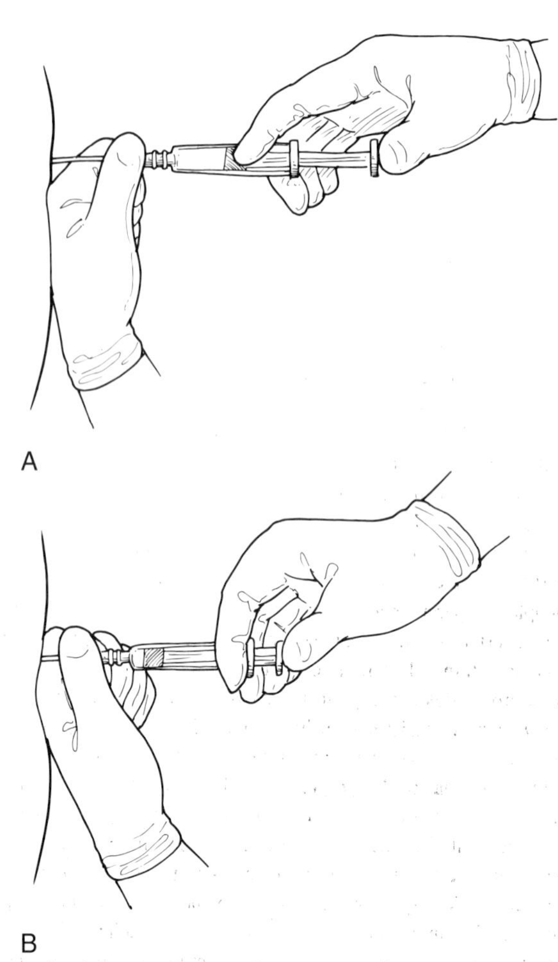

Fig 12–1 Loss of resistance technique during an epidural injection. **A**, Resistance present to the plunger of the syringe. **B**, Loss of resistance noted when needle tip is advanced into the epidural space.

Neuroaxial Compartment Injections

Midline Epidural Injection

CPT Codes

The Current Procedural Terminology codes for this procedure are 62310 (cervical or thoracic) and 62311 (lumbar).

A midline epidural injection is typically performed to treat or help diagnose primary discogenic pain. This technique has been used for decades to treat spinal pain and continues to be one of the standards in spinal procedures. Common levels performed range between the C6–7 to the L5–S1 level. This procedure is usually performed with the patient in the prone position under fluoroscopic guidance.

1. Locate the spinous processes of the vertebrae above and below the target level and mark the skin.
2. Mark the *inferior* border of the lamina of the most cephalad vertebrae and the *superior* border of the lamina of the most caudad vertebrae.
3. Scrub the skin with Betadine or Hibiclens and use sterile drapes in the field.
4. Anesthetize the skin, subcutaneous tissue, and interspinous ligaments with 1% lidocaine.
5. Advance an 18- or 20-gauge Tuohy needle through the interspinous ligament into the ligamentum flavum. (Figures 12–2 and 12–3)

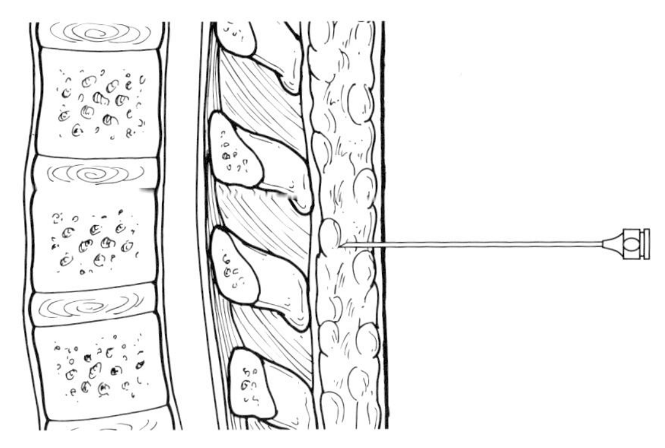

Fig 12–2 Epidural injection. The needle tip is placed initially through the skin and fat and advanced into the spinous ligaments.

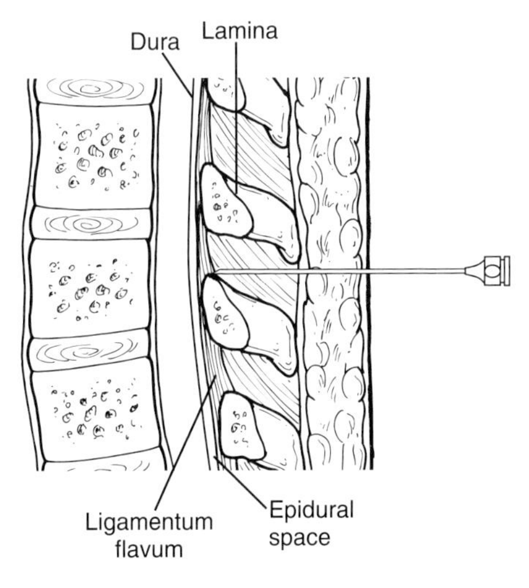

Fig 12–3 Epidural injection. The needle tip is advanced to the ligamentum flavum.

6. With the loss of resistance technique, the Tuohy needle is slowly and carefully advanced through the ligamentum flavum until the resistance on the syringe is lost and the epidural space is entered. (Figure 12–4)
7. Inject 3–5 cc of contrast to confirm proper needle placement and to avoid vascular uptake.
8. Change syringes, and inject a solution of corticosteroid and anesthetic, typically 5–10 cc of volume.

Take your time to mark the landmarks precisely.

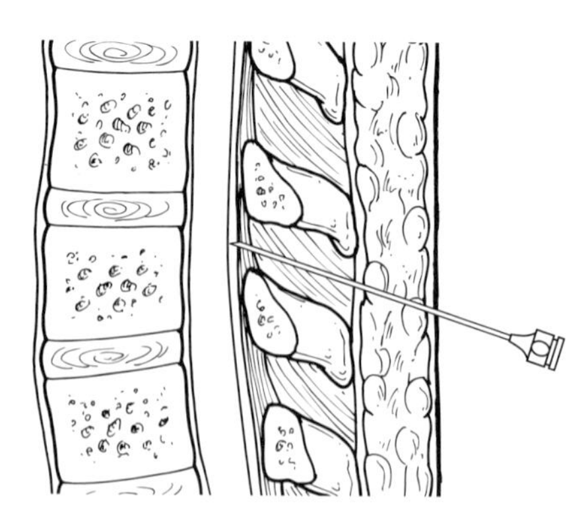

Fig 12–4 Epidural injection. The needle tip penetrates the ligamentum flavum and enters the epidural space.

Paramedian Epidural Approach (Figures 12–5 and 12–6)

CPT Codes

The Current Procedural Terminology codes for this procedure are 62310 (cervical or thoracic) and 62311 (lumbar).

As an alternative to the midline approach, some physicians prefer a paramedian approach to the epidural space. This injection is identical to the midline approach as noted previously, with the exception that the Tuohy needle enters the spine just lateral to the midline and is advanced through the paraspinal muscles to the cephalad border of the lamina. The needle tip is then gradually moved upward and advanced initially into the ligamentum flavum and then into the epidural space (Figure 12–7).

Transforaminal Epidural Injection

CPT Codes

The Current Procedural Terminology codes for this procedure are 64479 (cervical or thoracic—single level), 64480 (each additional level), 64483 (lumbar or sacral—single level), and 64484 (each additional level).

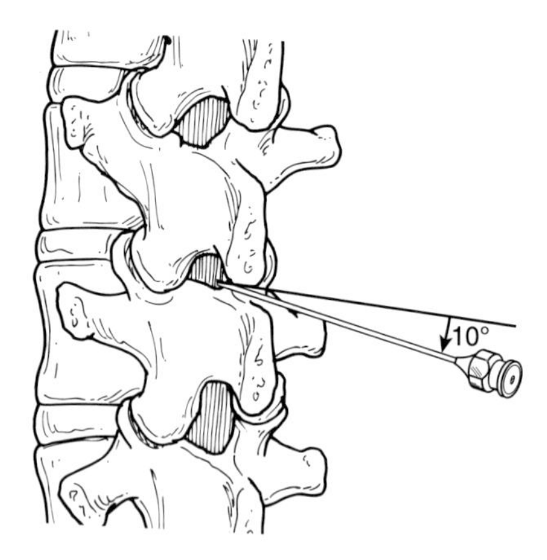

Fig 12–5 Lumbar paramedian epidural injection. Note the location of the needle tip adjacent to the midline.

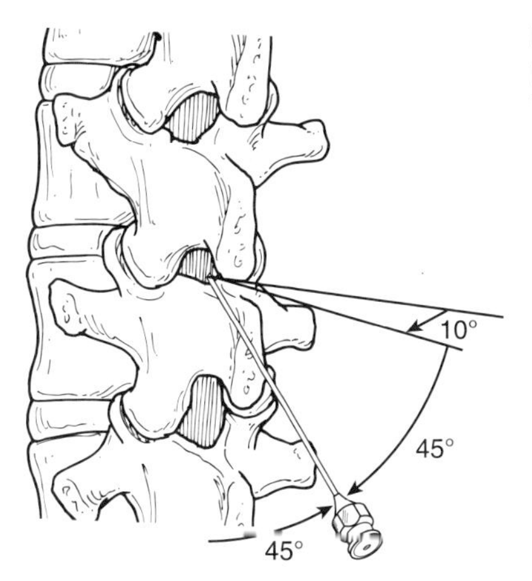

Fig 12–6 Epidural injection: lumbar paramedium epidural injection. Note the needle tip is advanced cephalad.

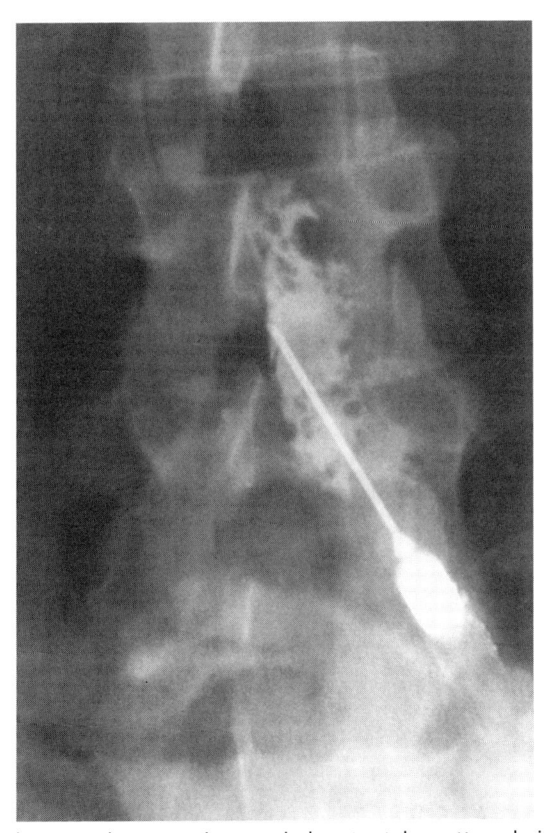

Fig 12–7 Lumbar x-ray demonstrating a typical contrast dye pattern during a paramedian epidural injection.

The most difficult epidural injection to perform is the transforaminal injection because of the tactile skills required to attain the correct needle trajectory for a successful block and the degree of difficulty interpreting the fluoroscopic image. This injection requires precise needle placement adjacent to the neuroforamen and is commonly performed to alleviate or diagnose radicular symptoms thought to be originating from the neuroaxial compartment of the spine (Figures 12–8 and 12–9). Cervical transforaminal epidural injections should be performed only by experienced physicians who are knowledgeable of the cervical anatomy and are aware of the serious complications associated with faulty technique.

The patient is placed in the prone position under fluoroscopic guidance.

1. The transverse processes above and below the desired target neuroforamen and the lateral margin of the lamina are marked on the skin. The C3–L5 neuroforamen are usually accessible with the patient in this prone position. Cervical injections may require a slight oblique tilt. Some physicians prefer an oblique approach to all levels except the S1. Identifying marks for the L5 transforaminal injection differ from the levels noted previously by replacing the lower transverse process mark

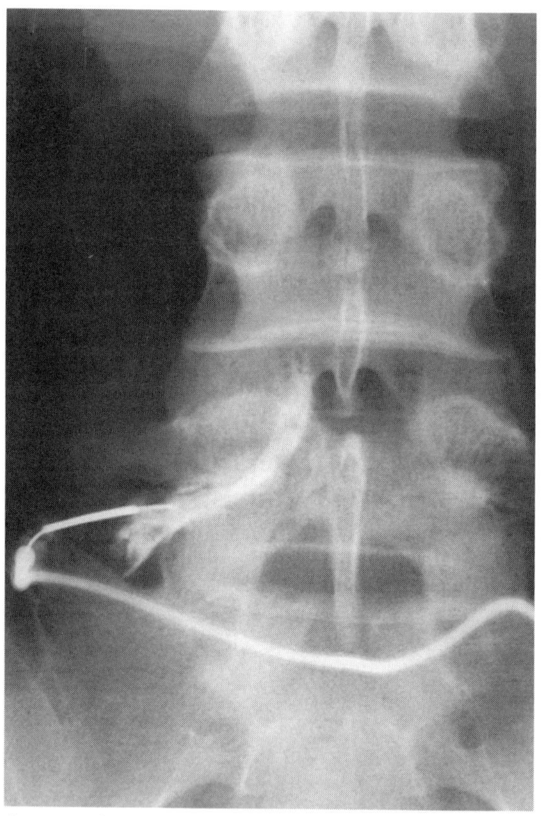

Fig 12–8 Lumbar x-ray demonstrating a typical contrast dye pattern during an L5 transforaminal epidural injection.

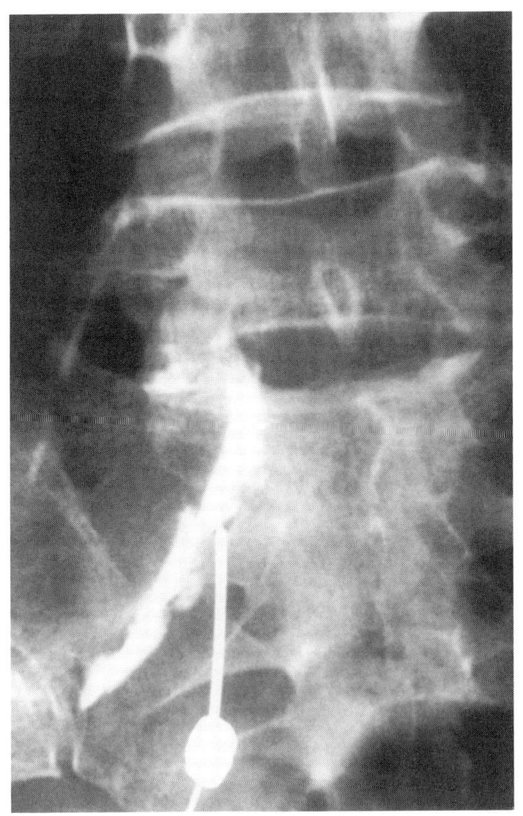

Fig 12–9 Lumbar x-ray demonstrating a typical contrast dye pattern during an S1 transforaminal epidural injection.

with the upper border of the sacrum. In addition, the S1 block is performed through the S1 foramen located on the dorsal sacrum.

2. The skin is scrubbed with Betadine or Hibiclens, and a sterile drape is applied to the field.
3. Three to five cubic centimeters of 1% lidocaine is injected into the skin, subcutaneous tissue, and muscle.
4. A 3½-inch 22- or 25-gauge spinal needle is inserted just below the inferior aspect of the pedicle *superior* to the exiting nerve root. If the S1 foramen is the target, the needle is advanced into this opening. Several changes in the needle trajectory are common.
5. Two to five cubic centimeters of contrast can be injected to verify needle placement and to prevent vascular injection.
6. Three to five cubic centimeters of a corticosteroid and anesthetic mixture can be injected.

Caudal Epidural Approach

CPT Code

The Current Procedural Terminology code for this procedure is 62311 (lumbar).

The use of caudal epidural steroid injections is limited to those patients with lower lumbosacral disc disease, mainly involving the L5–S1 and possibly the L4–5 segments. This approach has less risk of dural puncture because the dural sac typically terminates at the second sacral segment. The patient is placed in the prone position, and the procedure is performed under fluoroscopic guidance.

1. Palpate the sacral cornu and the sacral hiatus.
2. Scrub the skin with Betadine or Hibiclens and use sterile drapes in the field.
3. Anesthetize the skin and the subcutaneous tissue within the sacral hiatus with 1% lidocaine. Maintain one finger on the sacral hiatus as the anesthesia is injected and as the overlying skin expands.
4. With a 22- or 25-gauge spinal needle, insert the tip into the sacral hiatus at a 30-degree angle to the sacrum (Figure 12–10).
5. Once the needle has penetrated the sacral hiatus, slightly withdraw the needle and readvance parallel to the sacrum.
6. Advance the needle tip approximately 2 cm from the sacral hiatus.
7. Attach a 5-cc syringe to the spinal needle and slowly aspirate to check for blood or cerebrospinal fluid.
8. Inject 3–5 cc of contrast dye to confirm needle placement (Figure 12–11).
9. Change syringes and incrementally inject 10–20 cc of volume consisting of a 0.5% or 1% lidocaine and corticosteroid mix.

Z-Joint or Facet Joint Injections

Z-joint injections can be performed in the cervical, thoracic, or lumbar regions and are considered the "gold standard" for diagnosing posterior element pain. They may also be very effective in the treatment of this pain as well. Although difficult to isolate, one may suspect these joints as either the primary or secondary pain generator when a patient experiences unilateral or bilateral pain just lateral to midline, worse with extension and rotation. Frequently the z-joint is only one structure of several possibilities that may be causing pain within the spinal axis, and, therefore, injections directed toward these joints in these cases would be expected to give only partial pain relief. There are two injection methods when the z-joint is the suspected cause of

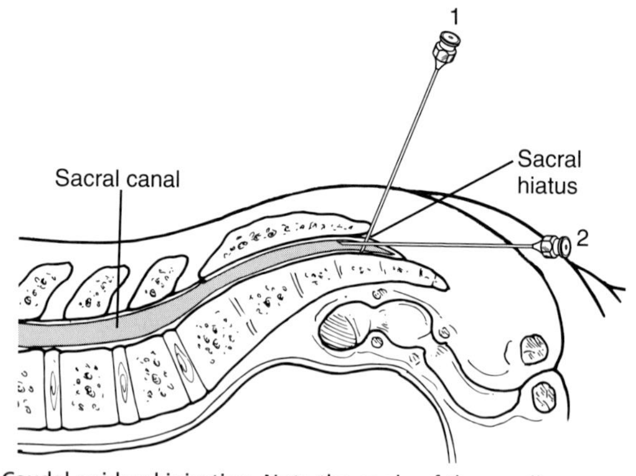

Fig 12–10 Caudal epidural injection. Note the angle of the needles.

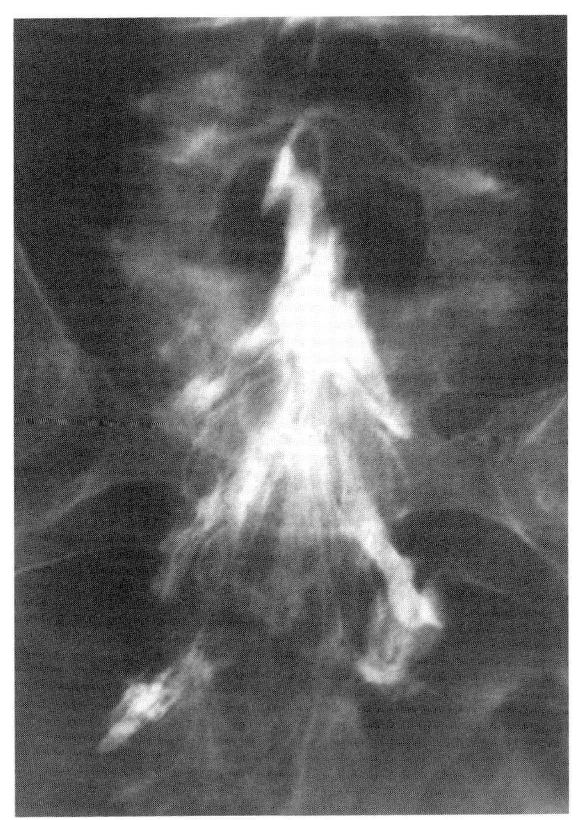

Fig 12–11 Lumbar x-ray demonstrating a typical contrast dye pattern during a caudal epidural injection.

pain, intra-articular and the diagnostic medial branch block (MBB) (facet joint nerve). Intra-articular injections deposit either an anesthetic or anesthetic-corticosteroid mixture into the joint. An MBB uses an anesthetic to temporarily anesthetize the nerve, thereby directly affecting the individual joint. Because of the dual innervation of these joints, two medial branches must be blocked to effectively anesthetize a single target joint. The diagnostic MBB is often performed as a prelude to a medial branch neurotomy.

Intra-Articular Z-Joint Injections

CPT Codes

The Current Procedural Terminology codes for this procedure are 64470 (cervical or thoracic—single level), 64472 (each additional level), 64475 (lumbar—single level), and 64476 (each additional level).

Intra-articular (IA) z or facet injections are commonly performed throughout the spinal axis. Variation in regional anatomy within the cervical, thoracic, or lumbar spine requires minor adjustments in technique and awareness of potential complications. IA z-joint injections require fluoroscopy to visualize each joint before injection. In general, these procedures are technically easy to perform compared with epidural injections but can be time consuming, especially when multiple joints are to be injected.

1. Place the patient in a prone–oblique position under fluoroscopy.
2. The T12–L1 through the L4–5 joints should be easy to identify with the patient in this position. If the L5–S1 joint is desired, the patient can be repositioned into a direct prone position. Cervical joint injections can be performed from a posterior or lateral position. Thoracic joint injections are performed with the patient in the prone position.
3. Mark the target joints on the skin.
4. Scrub the skin with Betadine or Hibiclens and use sterile drapes in the field.
5. Anesthetize the skin, subcutaneous tissue, and muscle at each target site.
6. Use a 22- or 25-gauge spinal needle and slowly advance the needle tip under fluoroscopy into the joint. It may require several adjustments to the needle trajectory before the needle is visualized and felt to enter the joint (Figure 12–12).
7. Inject 0.5–1 cc of contrast to confirm needle placement (Figures 12–13 and 12–14).
8. Aspirate the contrast and inject a mixture of 1% or 2% lidocaine and corticosteroid.

Medial Branch Blocks

CPT Codes

The Current Procedural Terminology codes for this procedure are 64470 (cervical or thoracic—single level), 64472 (each additional level), 64475 (lumbar—single level), and 64476 (each additional level).

A brief overview of the procedure is described here, but more detailed text can be found in other textbooks (Bogduk, 2004; Dreyfuss *et al.*, 2000).

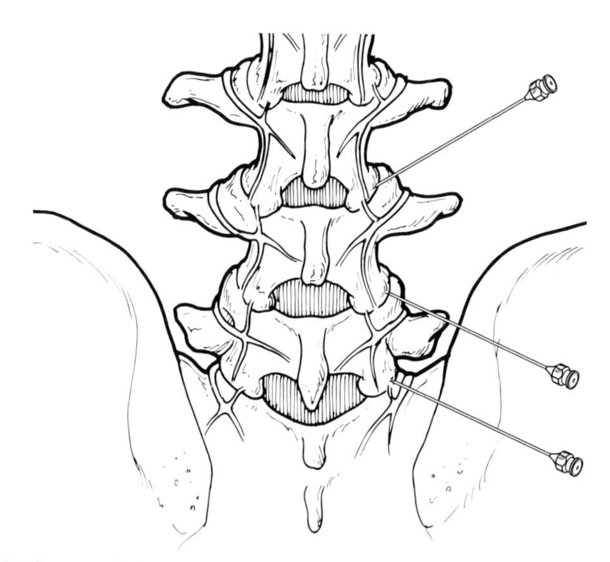

Fig 12–12 Diagram of the lumbar spine demonstrating needle placement for intra-articular lumbar facet injections.

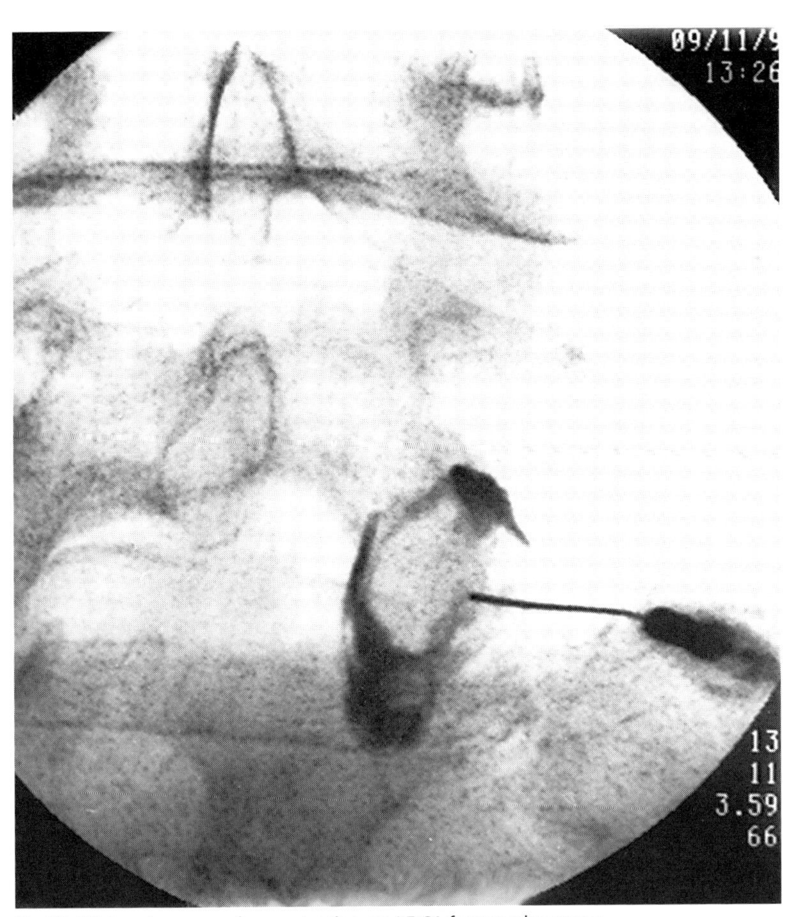

Fig 12–13 Lumbar x-ray demonstrating an L5-S1 facet arthrogram.

1. Place the patient in a prone position under fluoroscopic guidance. (For cervical, a posterior or lateral approach can be used.)
2. For lumbar blocks, two medial branch blocks are necessary for a single joint (i.e., L4–5 joint is affected when the L3 medial branch at the transverse process of L4 and the L4 medial branch at the transverse process of L5 is blocked) The target site for the needle tip is the L1–L4 blocks; the medial branch should be blocked at the junction of the superior articular process and the transverse process (Figure 12–15).

For thoracic blocks (T1–T4 and T9–T10), the skin entry point is directly over the target nerve, and the needle tip should be positioned at the superolateral aspect of the transverse process. For T5–8, the target area should also include an area just above and medial to the superolateral corner of the transverse process.

For cervical blocks (C3–6), the needle tip is inserted toward the center portion of the articular pillar (C7), and the needle tip is placed at the lateral aspect of the superior articular process.

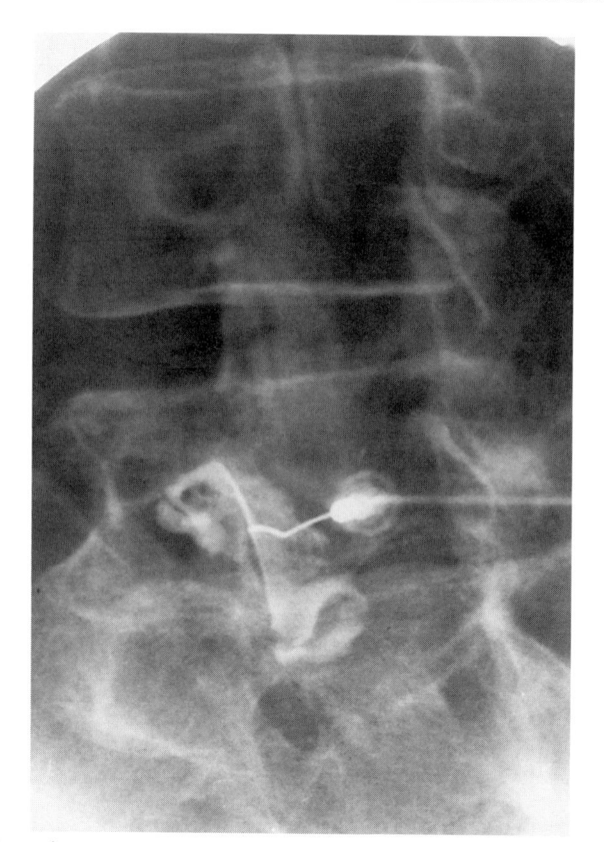

Fig 12–14 Lumbar x-ray demonstrating a lumbar facet arthrogram (oblique view).

3. Mark the target sites on the skin.
4. Scrub the skin with Betadine or Hibiclens and use sterile drapes in the field.
5. Anesthetize the skin, subcutaneous tissue, and muscle at each target site.
6. Use a 22- or 25-gauge spinal needle and slowly advance the needle tip under fluoroscopy to the target site.
7. Inject 0.1–0.2 cc of contrast.
8. Inject 0.3 cc of anesthetic (either 1% or 2% lidocaine).
9. The patient's response should be closely monitored and recorded.

SI Joint Injection

CPT Code

The Current Procedural Terminology code for this procedure is 27096 (sacroiliac joint injection).

Intra-articular sacroiliac joint injections are technically easy to perform with fluoroscopic guidance and with the patient in the prone position.

1. Mark the inferior third of the joint on the skin.
2. Scrub the skin with Betadine or Hibiclens and use sterile drapes in the field.
3. Anesthetize the skin and subcutaneous tissue over the site to be injected with 3–5 cc of 1% lidocaine.

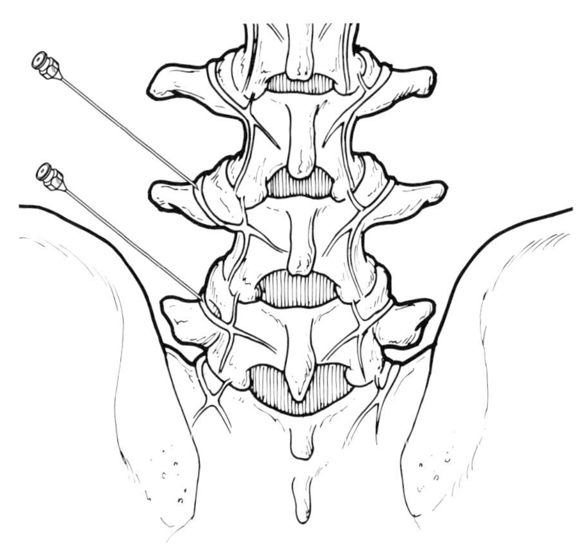

Fig 12–15 Diagram of the lumbar spine demonstrating needle placement for a medial branch block (MBB).

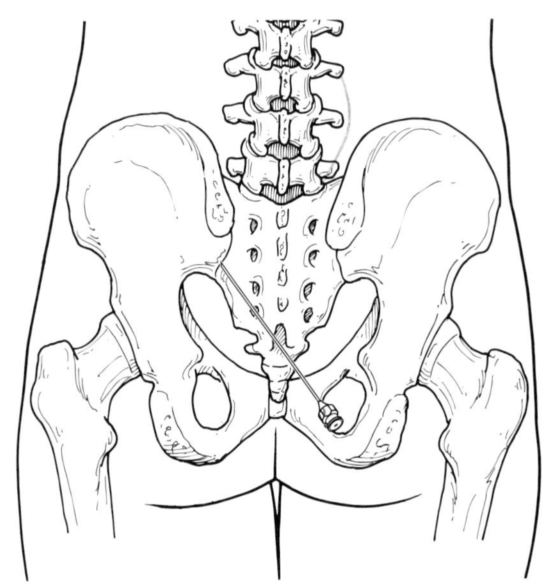

Fig 12–16 Diagram of the pelvis demonstrating needle placement in the sacroiliac joint.

4. Slowly advance a 3½-inch 22- or 25-gauge spinal needle under fluoroscopic guidance into the lower portion of the joint (Figure 12–16).
5. Inject contrast into the joint to confirm proper needle placement.
6. Inject a 5-cc solution of 1% lidocaine and corticosteroid.

The only reliable location to inject the SI joint is in the inferior third of the joint.

Conclusion

Spinal injections are useful procedures to assist in the diagnosis of painful spinal problems and to promote a higher level of function. These injections are useful when used within a broader framework of a spinal rehabilitation program. The specialist who chooses to perform spinal injections should be properly trained in the various procedures and be competent in patient selection and their knowledge of the regional anatomy. They should also be able to recognize and manage all potential complications that may occur from each procedure.

REFERENCES

Bogduk N., Ed. (2004). Practice Guidelines for Spinal Diagnostic and Treatment Procedures. International Spinal Injection Society, San Francisco, CA.

Botwin, K. P., Gruber, R. D., Bouchlas, C. G., *et al.* (2002). Fluoroscopically guided lumbar transforaminal epidural steroid injections in degenerative lumbar stenosis: An outcome study. *Am. J. Phys. Med. Rehabil.* **81(12),** 898–905.

Brouwers, P., Kottnik, E., Simon, M., and Prevo, R. L. (1991). A cervical anterior spinal artery syndrome after diagnostic blockade of the right C6 nerve root. *Pain* **91,** 397–399.

Derby, R., Kine, G., Saal, J., *et al.* (1992). Response to steroid and duration of radicular pain as predictors of surgical outcome. *Spine* **17,** 5176–5183.

Dreyfuss, P., Kaplan, M., and Dreyer, S. (2000). Zygapophyseal joint injection techniques in the spinal axis. *In* Pain Procedures in Clinical Practice. (T. A. Lennard, Ed.). 2nd ed. pp. 276–308. Hanley & Belfus, Philadelphia.

Houton, J. K., and Errico, T. J. (2002). Paraplegia after lumbosacral nerve root block; Report of three cases. *Spine J.* **2,** 70–75.

Kaplan, M., and Derby, R. J. (1998). Epidural corticosteroid injections: When, why, and how. *J. Musculoskel. Med.* **15,** 39–46.

Krames, E. S. (1999). Interventional pain management. Appropriate when less invasive therapies fail to provide adequate analgesia. *Med. Clin. North Am.* **83,** 787–788, vii–viii.

Tong, H. C., Williams, J. C., Haig, A. J., e*t al.* (2004). Predicting outcomes of transforaminal epidural injections for sciatica. *Spine J.* **4(5),** 605–606.

Index

Abscess, epidural, 185
Achilles retrocalcaneal bursa injection, 100–102
CPT code for, 100
examination findings for, 100
follow-up injections, 102
how and where to inject, 100, 101*f*
local anatomy for, 100
needle size/gauge for, 100
pitfalls/complications, 101
postinjection care, 102
Achilles tendon. *See also* Achilles retrocalcaneal bursa injection; Achilles tendonitis injection; Subcutaneous Achilles bursa injection
chondrotoxic corticosteroids risk to, 7
Achilles tendonitis injection, 77–79
CPT code for, 77
examination findings for, 77
follow-up injections, 79
how and where to inject, 77, 78*f*
local anatomy for, 77
needle size/gauge for, 77
pitfalls/complications, 79
postinjection care, 79
ACL. *See* Anterior cruciate ligament
Acromioclavicular joint injection, 19–21
CPT code for, 19
how and where to inject, 19, 20*f*
indications for, 19
needle size and gauge for, 19
pitfalls/complications of, 20
postinjection care, 21
Acupuncture, 172–177. *See also* Complimentary/alternative medicine
American interest in, 175, 176
chemotherapy-related nausea treatment, 175, 175*t*
conventional medicine's inclusion of, 176
evidence-based indications for, 175*t*
mechanism of action, 172, 173*f*, 174*f*, 175*f*, 175*t*
National Institutes of Health on, 175
potential risks, 176
Acute fracture, as contraindication for injection, 6*t*
Adrenalin administration
adverse patient reaction antidote, 5
emergency preparedness with, 3
Allergic reaction
as injection contraindication, 6*t*
spinal injection causing, 185
Ambu bag/mask, 3
Amenorrhea, corticosteroids side effect, 9
Amide anesthetics, 10, 10*t*
Anaphylaxis, injection causing, 5
Anatomical accuracy, 1, 2*t*. *See also* specific injection
Androgenic steroids, 9
glucocorticosteroids v., 8
Anesthetics, 10
amide, 10, 10*t*
common, 10*t*
ester, 10, 10*t*
interference with cardiovascular system, 11
needles for
skin injection, 12
soft tissue injection, 12
spinal injection, 12
side effects, 10
cardiovascular complications, 11
CNS complications, 11
toxicity to, 11, 186
hyaluronic acid, 12
vasoconstrictor agents, 11
Ankle joint injection, 47–49
CPT code for, 47
examination findings for, 47
follow-up injections, 49
how and where to inject, 48, 48*f*, 49*f*
local anatomy for, 47
needle size/gauge for, 47
pitfalls/complications, 48
postinjection care, 49
Anterior cruciate ligament (ACL), 2*t*, 167
Anterior tarsal tunnel. *See* Deep peroneal nerve injection
Anticoagulants, as contraindication for injection, 6*t*

Anti-inflammatory steroids, 9
- potencies, 9*t*

Antiseptics, skin, 13
Anxiety
- as contraindication for injection, 6*t*
- corticosteroids side effect, 9

Appetite increase, corticosteroids side effect, 9
Arthritis, glucocorticoids causing
- crystal -induced, 9

Aseptic technique
- equipment for, 2, 3*t*
- gloves for, 3, 3*t*
- septic injection risk v., 7
- skin antiseptics, 13

Aspirates
- bloody, 88
- categories of, 2*t*
- cloudy, 88
- evidence of infection, 7
- frank blood, 2*t*

Aspirating
- needles for, 12
- tip for, 3

Atrophy, subcutaneous, 6
- glucocorticoids causing, 9

Band-Aids, 13
- spinal injections, 186*t*

Benefit/risk profile (for injection), 1
Betamethasone, anti-inflammatory effect of, 9*t*
Bicipital tendinitis injection, 62–66
- CPT code for, 62
- examination findings for, 64
- follow-up injections, 66
- how and where to inject, 64, 65*f*
- local anatomy for, 64
- needle size/gauge for, 64
- pitfalls/complications, 64
- postinjection care, 66

Bleeding
- gastrointestinal, 9
- injection causing, 6
- spinal injection causing, 185

Blood
- frank, 2*t*
- post-injection elevated leukocyte count, 7

Bone
- cartilage attrition, 9
- fractured, as contraindication for injection, 6*t*
- necrotic, as corticosteroid side effect, 9
- osteopathic manual medicine, 156
- osteoporosis, 9

Botox, 160
Botulinum toxin injection, 156
- clinical uses of, 162
- CPT code for, 162
- examination findings for, 163
- how and where to inject, 164, 164*f*
- indications for, 163
- mechanism of action, 156
- medications to inject, 163
- needle size/gauge for, 163
- overdosing, 161
- pitfalls/complications, 164
- poor injection technique, 161
- postinjection care, 164
- potential risks, 161
- reactions to medication, 161

Bruising, injection causing, 6
Bupivicaine, 10*t*, 11*t*, 182
Bursa injection
- Achilles retrocalcaneal, 100–102
  - CPT code for, 100
  - examination findings for, 100
  - follow-up injections, 102
  - how and where to inject, 100, 101*f*
  - local anatomy for, 100
  - needle size/gauge for, 100
  - pitfalls/complications, 101
  - postinjection care, 102
- Achilles subcutaneous
  - CPT code for, 102
  - examination findings for, 102
  - follow-up injections, 104
  - how and where to inject, 103, 103*f*, 104*f*
  - local anatomy for, 103
  - needle size/gauge for, 103
  - pitfalls/complications, 103
  - postinjection care, 103
- ischial, 92–95
  - CPT code for, 92
  - examination findings for, 93
  - follow-up injections, 95
  - how and where to inject, 93, 94*f*
  - local anatomy for, 93
  - needle size/gauge for, 93
  - pitfalls/complications, 93
  - postinjection care, 93
- olecranon, 20–87
  - CPT code for, 87
  - examination findings for, 88
  - follow-up injections, 90
  - how and where to inject, 88, 89*f*
  - local anatomy for, 88
  - needle size/gauge for, 88
  - pitfalls/complications, 89
  - postinjection care, 90
- pes anserine, 95–97
  - CPT code for, 69
  - examination findings for, 95
  - follow-up injections, 97
  - how and where to inject, 96, 96*f*, 97*f*
  - local anatomy for, 95
  - needle size/gauge for, 95
  - pitfalls/complications, 96
  - postinjection care, 96
- subacromial (subdeltoid), 85–87
  - CPT code for, 85

examination findings for, 85
follow-up injections, 87
how and where to inject, 86, 86*f*, 87*f*
local anatomy for, 86
needle size/gauge for, 86
pitfalls/complications, 87
postinjection care, 87
trochanteric, 90–92
CPT code for, 90
examination findings for, 90
follow-up injections, 92
how and where to inject, 85, 91, 91*f*
local anatomy for, 90
needle size/gauge for, 90
pitfalls/complications, 91
postinjection care, 91
Bursitis injection. *See* Bursa injection; Iliotibial band tendinitis injection

Calcification, glucocorticoids causing, 9
CAM. *See* Complimentary/alternative medicine
Cardiac arrest, injection causing, 5
Cardiopulmonary resuscitation (CPR), 5. *See also* Respiratory depression
equipment for, 186*t*
Cardiovascular system
anesthesia's interference with, 11
spinal injection risks to, 185
Cardioversion equipment, spinal injection requiring, 186*t*
Carpal joint injection. *See* First carpometacarpal joint injection
Carpal tunnel injection. *See* Median nerve injection (at wrist)
Carpometacarpal joint injection. *See* First carpometacarpal joint injection
Cartilage, attrition of, glucocorticoids causing, 9
Cataracts, corticosteroids side effect, 9
Caudal epidural injection, 190*f*, 191*f*, 192*f*, 193
Central nervous system (CNS), 11
acupuncture influencing, 176
anesthetic toxicity to, 11, 186
hyaluronic acid, 12
vasoconstrictor agents, 11
Cervical stellate ganglion blocks, 181*f*, 182*f*
CPT code for, 180
"Chalk," injection causing, 7
Chemotherapy-related nausea, acupuncture's value for, 175, 175*t*
Children under eighteen years old, as contraindication for injection, 6*t*
Chloroprocaine, 10*t*
Chondrotoxic drugs, 7
Achilles tendon risk from, 7
Circulatory collapse, injection causing, 5. *See also* Cardiopulmonary resuscitation
Clostridium botulinum, 160
CNS. *See* Central nervous system
Complex regional pain syndrome (CRPS), 178, 179
Type I diagnostic criteria, 179*t*
Type II diagnostic criteria, 180*t*
Complimentary/alternative medicine (CAM), 176. *See also* Acupuncture
Chinese traditional, 172
osteopathic manual medicine, 156
Congestive heart failure, corticosteroids side effect, 9
Corticosteroids. *See also* Glucocorticosteroids
amenorrhea from, 9
chondrotoxic, 7
risk to Achilles tendon from, 7
classification of, 9
gastrointestinal bleeding from, 9
gluco-, androgenic steroids v., 8
gluco-, cosmetic changes from, 9
hydrocortisone, 9*t*
long-term use side effects, 9
reactions to, spinal injections causing, 185
salt retaining steroids, 9
short-term use side effects, 9
systemic, 9
spinal injections, 186*t*
"steroid trail," 9
Cortisol, 9
anti-inflammatory effect of, 9*t*
Cortisone, anti-inflammatory effect of, 9*t*
Cosmetic changes, glucocorticoids causing, 9
CPR. *See* Cardiopulmonary resuscitation
CPT. *See* Current procedural terminology
CRPS. *See* Complex regional pain syndrome
Current procedural terminology (CPT). *See specific injection site*
Cushingoid appearance, corticosteroids side effect, 9

De Quervain's tenosynovitis injection, 61–62
CPT code for, 61
examination findings for, 61
follow-up injections, 62
how and where to inject, 62, 63*f*
local anatomy for, 61
needle size/gauge for, 61
pitfalls/complications, 62
Death, as patient reaction (to injection), 5
Deep peroneal nerve injection, 145
CPT code for, 145
examination findings for, 145
follow-up injections, 148
how and where to inject, 146, 147*f*
local anatomy for, 146
needle size/gauge for, 146
pitfalls/complications, 146
postinjection care, 148

Depigmentation, 6, 89
glucocorticoids causing, 9
Dexamethasone, anti-inflammatory effect of, 9*t*
Dextrose-based solution, 168*t*
Diabetic patient, as contraindication for injection, 6*t*
Diathermy, 156
Digital nerve block injection. *See* Lower extremity digital nerve block injection
Disposable plastic airways, 3
Dosage problem, 4
Dystonia, 160

Edema, injection causing, 5
Elbow joint injection
CPT for, 23
examination findings prior to, 24
follow-up injections, 26
how and where to inject, 24, 25*f*
local anatomy, 23–26
needle size/gauge for, 24
pitfalls/complications of, 26
Electrotherapy, intradiscal, 187
Epidural injection
abscess/hematoma from, 185
caudal, 190*f*, 191*f*, 192*f*, 193
paramedian, 190
transforaminal, 190
Epinephrine, contraindication for, 34
Epi-Pen, 3
reduced risk with, 5
Ester anesthetics, 10, 10*t*
Estrogenic steroids, 9
Etidocaine, 10*t*, 11*t*

Facet joint spinal injection, 193*f*, 194, 194*f*, 195*f*, 196*f*, 197*f*
FDA. *See* Food and Drug Administration
Femoral nerve injection, 137–139
CPT code for, 137
examination findings for, 137
follow-up injections, 139
how and where to inject, 136*f*, 138*f*, 139*f*, 138
local anatomy for, 137
needle size/gauge for, 137
pitfalls/complications, 139
postinjection care, 139
Fever, injection causing, 7
First carpometacarpal joint injection, 31–34
CPT for, 31
examination findings prior to, 32
how and where to inject, 32, 33*f*
indications for, 31
needle size/gauge, 32
pitfalls/complications of, 32
postinjection care, 34
Fluoroscopy, c-arm, spinal injections requiring, 186*t*
Flushing
corticosteroid side effect, 9
injection causing, 5
spinal injection causing, 185
Food and Drug Administration (FDA)
botox, 160
Fracture, acute, as contraindication for injection, 6*t*
Frank blood, 2*t*
Frank pus, 2*t*

Gastrointestinal bleeding, 9
Glaucoma, corticosteroid side effect, 9
Glenohumeral joint injection, 15
anterior approach to, 16, 16*f*, 17*f*
CPT code for, 15
follow-up injections, 18
local anatomy, 16
needle size/gauge, 16
pitfalls and complications of, 18
posterior approach to, 17, 17*f*, 18*f*
postinjection care, 18
Gloves
aseptic technique requiring, 3, 3*t*
sterile and nonsterile, 13
Glucocorticosteroids, 8. *See also* Corticosteroids
androgenic steroids v., 8
anti-inflammatory effect of, 8, 9*t*
cartilage attrition from, 9
short-term use side effects, 9
subcutaneous atrophy from, 6, 9, 89
Gout, 89

Hair loss, glucocorticoids causing, 9
Headache
diagnostic for, 111
migraine, acupuncture for, 175*t*
spinal injection causing, 185
Heat with ultrasound, 156
Hematoma, spinal injection causing epidural, 185
Hepatitis B, vaccination for, 3
Hip joint injections, 39–43
CPT code for, 39
examination findings for, 39
follow-up injections, 43
how and where to inject
anterior approach, 40, 41*f*
lateral approach, 42*f*
local anatomy for, 40
needle size/gauge for, 40
pitfalls/complications, 40
postinjection care, 42
Horner's syndrome, as cervical stellate ganglion block feature, 182
Hyaluronic acid, CNS toxicity from, 12
Hydrocortisone, anti-inflammatory effect of, 9*t*

Hyperglycemia, 9
Hyperlipidemia, 9
Hypersensitivity, as contraindication for injection, 6*t*
Hypertension, corticosteroid side effect, 9
Hypothalamic-pituitary-adrenal axis, corticosteroids influencing, 9

Ice pack, 4, 156
IDET. *See* Intradiscal electrotherapy
Iliohypogastric nerve block injection, 127–129
  CPT code for, 127
  examination findings for, 127
  follow-up injections, 129
  how and where to inject, 127, 128*f*
  local anatomy for, 127
  needle size/gauge for, 127
  pitfalls/complications, 129
  postinjection care, 129
Iliotibial band tendinitis injection, 79–82
  CPT code for, 79
  examination findings for, 80
  how and where to inject, 80, 81*f*
  local anatomy for, 80
  needle size/gauge, 80
  pitfalls/complications, 80
  postinjection care, 81
Ilioinguinal nerve block injection, 129–131
  CPT code for, 129
  examination findings for, 129
  follow-up injections, 131
  how and where to inject, 130, 130*f*, 131*f*
  local anatomy for, 130
  needle size/gauge for, 129
  pitfalls/complications, 130
  postinjection care, 131
Immunocompromised patient, as contraindication for injection, 6*t*
Infection
  as contraindication for injection, 6*t*
  control of, aseptic technique, 2, 3*t*
    equipment for, 2, 3*t*
    gloves for, 3, 3*t*
    septic injection risk v., 7
    skin antiseptics, 13
  risk of, from injection, 7
Inflammation
  anti-inflammatory steroids, 9
    potencies, 9*t*
  glucocorticosteroids v., 8, 9*t*
Infrapatellar tendinitis injection, 82–84
  CPT codes for, 82
  examination findings for, 82
  follow-up injections, 84
  how and where to inject, 83, 83*f*
  local anatomy for, 82
  needle size/gauge for, 82
  pitfalls/complications, 84
  postinjection care, 84
Injection. *See* Pain injections; *specific anatomical site*
Intercarpal joint, 29–31
  CPT code for, 29
Intercarpal joint injection
  how and where to inject, 30, 30*f*, 31*f*
  needle size/gauge for, 30
  pitfalls/complications of, 30
  postinjection care, 30
International Spinal Injection Society (ISIS), 185
Interphalangeal joint injection, 34–36
  CPT for, 34
  examination findings prior to, 34
  follow-up injections, 36
  how and where to inject, 35, 35*f*, 36*f*
  indications for, 34
  local anatomy, 35
  medications to inject, 34
  needle size/gauge for, 35
  pitfalls/complications of, 36
Intertarsal joint injection, 53–55
  CPT code for, 53
  examination findings for, 53
  follow-up injections, 55
  how and where to inject, 54, 54*f*
  local anatomy for, 53
  needle size/gauge for, 53
  pitfalls/complications, 55
  postinjection care, 55
Intra-articular z-joint spinal injection, 198*f*, 195
Intradiscal electrotherapy (IDET), 187
Intubation equipment, spinal injection requiring, 186*t*
Ischial bursa injection, 92–95
  CPT code for, 92
  examination findings for, 93
  follow-up injections, 95
  how and where to inject, 93, 94*f*
  local anatomy for, 93
  needle size/gauge for, 93
  pitfalls/complications, 93
  postinjection care, 93
ISIS. *See* International Spinal Injection Society

Joint. *See also specific joint*
  chondrotoxic corticosteroid risk to, 7
  prosthetic, 6*t*
  sclerotherapy, 166

Knee joint injection, 43–46
  CPT code for, 43
  examination findings for, 43
  follow-up injections, 46
  how and where to inject
    lateral approach, 44, 45*f*
    medial approach, 44, 46*f*
  local anatomy for, 44
  needle size/gauge for, 44

Knee joint injection (*Continued*)
- pitfalls/complications, 44
- postinjection care, 46

Lateral antebrachial cutaneous nerve injection, 114–118
- CPT code for, 114
- examination findings for, 116
- follow-up injections, 118
- how and where to inject, 117, 117*f*, 118*f*
- local anatomy for, 116
- needle size/gauge for, 116
- pitfalls/complications, 117
- postinjection care, 118

Lateral epicondylitis, 66–68
- CPT code for, 66
- examination findings for, 66
- follow-up injections, 68
- how and where to inject, 67, 67*f*, 68*f*
- local anatomy for, 67
- needle size/gauge for, 67
- pitfalls/complications, 67
- postinjection care, 68

Lateral femoral cutaneous nerve injection, 131–134
- CPT code for, 131
- examination findings for, 132
- follow-up injections, 134
- how and where to inject, 132, 133*f*
- local anatomy for, 132
- needle size/gauge for, 132
- pitfalls/complications, 132
- postinjection care, 134

Leukocyte count, post-injection elevated, 7

Lidocaine, 10*t*, 11*t*, 168*t*
- spinal injection with, 186*t*

Loss of resistance technique (spinal injection), 187, 188*f*, 189*f*, 190*f*

Lower extremity digital nerve block injection, 153–155
- CPT code for, 153
- examination findings for, 153
- follow-up injections, 155
- how and where to inject, 154, 154*f*
- local anatomy for, 153
- needle size/gauge for, 153
- pitfalls/complications, 155
- postinjection care, 155

Lumbar sympathetic blocks, 183*f*
- CPT code for, 182

Magnetic Resonance Imaging (MRI)
- glenohumeral joint, 18
- prolotherapy patient selection diagnostic, 167, 184
- spinal injection patient selection diagnostic, 184

Marcaine, spinal injection with, 186*t*

Massage, 156

MBB. *See* Medial branch block

Medial antebrachial cutaneous nerve injection, 113–114
- CPT code for, 113
- examination findings for, 113
- follow-up injections, 114
- how and where to inject, 114, 115*f*, 116*f*
- local anatomy for, 114
- needle size/gauge for, 114
- pitfalls/complications, 114
- postinjection care, 114

Medial branch block (MBB), 194, 196. *See also* Spinal injections
- procedure for, 196, 199*f*

Medial epicondylitis injection, 69–71
- CPT code for, 69
- examination findings for, 69
- follow-up injections, 71
- how and where to inject, 69, 70*f*
- local anatomy for, 69
- needle size/gauge for, 69
- pitfalls/complications for, 70
- postinjection care, 71

Median nerve injection (at wrist), 121–124
- CPT code for, 121
- examination findings for, 121
- follow-up injections, 124
- how and where to inject, 122, 123*f*
- local anatomy for, 122
- needle size/gauge for, 122
- pitfalls/complications, 122

Medication, 8. *See also specific type*
- allergic reaction to, 6*t*, 185
- anesthetic toxicity, 10, 11*t*
  - dosage reduction v., 11
- dosage problem, 4
- selection problem, 4

Mepivacaine, 10*t*, 11*t*

Meralgia paresthetica injection. *See* Lateral femoral cutaneous nerve injection

Metacarpal joint injection. *See* First carpometacarpal joint injection

Metatarsophalangeal joint injection, 55–57
- CPT code for, 55
- examination findings for, 55
- follow-up injections, 57
- how and where to inject, 56, 56*f*, 57*f*
- local anatomy for, 56
- needle size/gauge for, 56
- pitfalls/complications, 56
- postinjection care, 57

Methylprednisolone, anti-inflammatory effect of, 9*t*

Mood swings, 9

MRI. *See* Magnetic Resonance Imaging; Magnetic resonance imaging

Muscle. *See also specific muscle site*
- myofascial pain, 156
- weakness, 9

Musculocutaneous nerve injection, 108–110
CPT code for, 108
examination findings for, 108
follow-up injections, 110
how and where to inject, 109, 109*f*, 110*f*
local anatomy for, 108
needle size/gauge for, 108
pitfalls/complications, 110
postinjection care, 110
Myofascial pain, 156
Myopathy, corticosteroids side effect, 9

National Institutes of Health (NIH), on acupuncture, 175
Nausea and vomiting, acupuncture for postoperative, 175, 175*t*
Needles. *See also* Acupuncture; *specific injection site*
accuracy for placing, 1, 2*t*
aspirating, 12
commonly used, 12
size of, 4
skin injection, 12
soft tissue injection, 12
spinal injection, 12
Nerve. *See also* Spinal injections; Transcutaneous electrical nerve stimulation; *specific nerve*
damage, injection causing, 6
neuroaxial compartment injections, 188
stimulator, 109
NIH. *See* National Institutes of Health

Obturator nerve injection, 134–137
CPT code for, 134
examination findings for, 134
follow-up injections, 137
how and where to inject, 135
local anatomy for, 135
needle size/gauge for, 135
pitfalls/complications, 135
postinjection care, 135
Occipital nerve injection, 112f, 110–113
CPT code for, 110
examination findings for, 111
follow-up injections, 113
how and where to inject, 112, 112*f*
local anatomy for, 111
greater occipital, 111
lesser occipital, 111
needle size/gauge for, 111
pitfalls/complications, 113
postinjection care, 113
Olecranon bursa injection, 20–87
CPT code for, 87
examination findings for, 88
follow-up injections, 90
how and where to inject, 88, 89*f*
local anatomy for, 88
needle size/gauge for, 88
pitfalls/complications, 89
postinjection care, 90
Osteopathic manual medicine, 156
Osteoporosis, corticosteroids side effect, 9

Pain flare, postinjection, 6
Pain injections (general). *See also specific injection site*
benefit/risk profile prior to, 1
equipment for, 2, 3*t*
five rules of, 1
performing, 3
post injection care, 4
problems/issues of, 4
adverse patient reactions, 5, 6
contraindications to, 6*t*
poor technique, 5
protecting patient and self during, 3
supplies, 12
tip for, 3
Pancreatitis, corticosteroids side effect, 9
Paramedian epidural approach, 190
"Peppering" technique, 67
Peroneal nerve injection. *See* Deep peroneal nerve injection
Pes anserine bursa injection, 95–97
CPT code for, 69
examination findings for, 95
follow-up injections, 97
how and where to inject, 96, 96*f*, 97*f*
local anatomy for, 95
needle size/gauge for, 95
pitfalls/complications, 96
postinjection care, 96
Plantar fasciitis injection, 74–76
CPT code for, 74
examination findings for, 74
follow-up injections, 76
how and where to inject, 75, 75*f*, 76*f*
local anatomy for, 75
needle size/gauge for, 75
pitfalls/complications, 76
postinjection care, 76
Pneumothorax, risk of, 4
Postoperative nausea, acupuncture's value for, 175, 175*t*
Prednisolone, anti-inflammatory effect of, 9*t*
Prednisone, anti-inflammatory effect of, 9*t*
Prepatellar bursa injection, 97–99
CPT code for, 97
examination findings for, 98
follow-up injections, 99
how and where to inject, 98, 98*f*, 99*f*
local anatomy for, 98
needle size/gauge for, 98
pitfalls/complications, 99
postinjection care, 99

Procaine, 10*t*
Prolotherapy, 156–158
  contraindications to, 168*t*
  history of, 166
  injection sites, 168, 169*f*
  injection technique, 168
  mechanism of action/clinical effectiveness, 166
  patient selection, 167
  proliferative solutions, 167, 168*t*
Prosthetic joint, injections contraindicated for, 6*t*
Pus, frank, 2*t*

Radial nerve injection (at elbow), 118–121
  CPT code for, 118
  examination findings for, 119
  follow-up injections, 121
  how and where to inject, 119, 120*f*
  local anatomy for, 119
  needle size/gauge for, 119
  pitfalls/complications, 119
  postinjection care, 121
Rash, injection causing, 5
Regenerative injection therapy (RIT), 166. *See also* Prolotherapy
Respiratory depression. *See also* Cardiopulmonary resuscitation
  disposable plastic airways, 3
  injection causing, 5
Risk/benefit profile, 1
RIT. *See* Regenerative injection therapy
Rotator cuff tendinitis injection, 71–74
  CPT code for, 71
  examination findings for, 72
  follow-up injections, 74
  how and where to inject, 72, 73*f*
  local anatomy for, 72
  needle size/gauge for, 72
  pitfalls/complications, 73
  postinjection care, 74

Salt retaining steroids, 9
Saphenous nerve block injection, 139–142
  CPT code for, 140
  examination findings for, 140
  follow-up injections, 142
  how and where to inject, 141, 141*f*, 142*f*
    at ankle, 141
    at knee, 141
  local anatomy for, 140
  needle size/gauge for, 140
  pitfalls/complications, 141
  postinjection care, 142
Sclerotherapy, 166
Sepsis, injection causing, 7
Serous fluid, 2*t*
SI joint injection, procedure for, 198
Skin
  anesthesia, 12
  antiseptics for, 13
  depigmentation of, 6, 9, 89
  itchy, 5
  marker, 13
  rash, 5
Soreness, injection site, spinal injection causing, 185
Spasticity, 156
Speeds test, 64
Spinal injections, 184–200. *See also* Sympathetic injections
  anatomy, 187
  caudal epidural approach, 190*f*, 191*f*, 192*f*, 193
  equipment for, 185, 186*t*
  facet joint, 193*f*, 194, 194*f*, 195*f*, 196*f*, 197*f*
  loss of resistance technique, 187, 188*f*, 189*f*, 190*f*
  medial branch blocks, 194, 196
    procedure for, 196, 199*f*
  neuroaxial compartment injections, 188
  paramedian epidural approach, 190
  patient selection for, 184
  potential complications of, 185
  SI joint injection, 198
  specialists for, 185
  transforaminal epidural, 190
  z-joint, 193*f*, 194, 194*f*, 195*f*, 196*f*, 197*f*
    intra-articular, 195, 198*f*
Spray and stretch technique, 156
Stenosing flexor tenosynovitis. *See* Trigger finger injection
Stenosing tenosynovitis. *See* De Quervain's tenosynovitis injection
Sterile drapes, 13
Sternoclavicular joint injection, 21–23
  CPT code for, 21
  examination findings prior to, 21
  how and where to inject, 22, 22*f*, 23*f*
  indications for, 21
  local anatomy, 22
  needle size/gauge for, 22
  pitfalls/complications of, 23
  postinjection care, 23
"Steroid trail," 9
Subacromial bursa injection, 85–87
  CPT code for, 85
  examination findings for, 85
  follow-up injections, 87
  how and where to inject, 86, 86*f*, 87*f*
  local anatomy for, 86
  needle size/gauge for, 86
  pitfalls/complications, 87
  postinjection care, 87
Subcutaneous Achilles bursa injection, 102–104
  CPT code for, 102
  examination findings for, 102
  follow-up injections, 104

how and where to inject, 103, 103*f*, 104*f*
local anatomy for, 103
needle size/gauge for, 103
pitfalls/complications, 103
postinjection care, 103
Subdeltoid bursa injection. *See* Subacromial bursa injection
Subtalar joint injection, 49–53
CPT code for, 49
examination findings for, 50
follow-up injections, 53
how and where to inject, 50
lateral approach, 51, 52*f*
medial approach, 50, 51*f*
local anatomy for, 50
needle size/gauge for, 50
pitfalls/complications, 52
postinjection care, 52
Superficial peroneal ankle nerve injection, 148–150
CPT code for, 148
examination findings for, 148
follow-up injections, 150
how and where to inject, 149, 149*f*, 150*f*
local anatomy for, 149
needle size/gauge for, 149
pitfalls/complications, 150
postinjection care, 150
Superficial peroneal nerve injection (at ankle), 148–150
CPT code for, 148
examination findings for, 148
follow-up injections, 150
how and where to inject, 149*f*, 150*f*, 149
local anatomy for, 149
needle size/gauge for, 149
pitfalls/complications, 150
postinjection care, 150
Suprascapular nerve injection, 105–108
CPT code for, 105
examination findings for, 106
follow-up injections, 108
how and where to inject, 106, 107*f*
local anatomy for, 106
needle size/gauge for, 106
pitfalls/complications, 106
postinjection care, 106
Sural nerve block injection, 150–153
CPT code for, 151
examination findings for, 151
follow-up injections, 153
how and where to inject, 151, 152*f*
local anatomy for, 151
needle size/gauge for, 151
pitfalls/complications, 153
postinjection care, 153
Sympathetic injections, 178–183. *See also* Spinal injections
anatomy, 178
cervical stellate ganglion blocks, 180, 181*f*, 182*f*
CPT code for, 180
complex regional pain syndrome, 179, 179*t*, 180*t*
lumbar sympathetic blocks, 182, 183*f*
CPT code for, 182
patient selection for, 179*t*, 180, 180*t*
thoracic (paravertebral sympathetics), 182
Synasal, 166
Syncope, injection causing, 5
Syringes, 13

Tachycardia, corticosteroids side effect, 9
Tarsal tunnel injection. *See* Tibial nerve injection
TCM. *See* Traditional Chinese Medicine
Temporomandibular joint (TMJ) injection, 36–39, 167
CPT code for, 36
examination findings for, 37
follow-up injections, 39
how and where to inject, 37
local anatomy for, 37
needle size/gauge size for, 37
pitfalls/complications of, 38
post injection care, 39
prolotherapy for, 166
TENS. *See* Transcutaneous electrical nerve stimulation
Tetracaine, 10*t*
Thoracic (paravertebral sympathetics) injections, 182
Tibial nerve injection, 142–145
CPT code for, 142
examination findings for, 143
follow-up injections, 145
how and where to inject, 143, 144*f*
local anatomy for, 143
needle size/gauge for, 143
pitfalls/complications, 145
postinjection care, 145
TMJ. *See* Temporomandibular joint injection
Traditional Chinese Medicine (TCM), 172
Transcutaneous electrical nerve stimulation (TENS), 156
Transforaminal epidural, 190
Trauma, injection contraindicated for, 6*t*
Triamcinolone, anti-inflammatory effect of, 9*t*
Trigger finger injection (stenosing flexor tenosynovitis), 58–60
CPT code for, 58
examination findings for, 58–59
follow-up injections, 60–61
pitfalls/complications, 60
postinjection care, 60

Trigger point injection, 156–159
CPT code for, 157
examination findings for, 158
follow-up injections, 159
how and where to inject, 158, 159*f*
indications for, 157
mechanism of action, 156
medications to inject, 158
needle size/gauge for, 158
pitfalls/complications, 158
postinjection care, 159
potential risks, 157
trigger points, 156
Trochanteric bursa injection, 90–92
CPT code for, 90
examination findings for, 90
follow-up injections, 92
how and where to inject, 91, 91*f*
local anatomy for, 90
needle size/gauge for, 90
pitfalls/complications, 91
postinjection care, 91
Tubing, 13
Turbid fluid, 2*t*

Ulnar nerve injection, 124–126
CPT code for, 124
examination findings for, 124
follow-up injections, 126
how and where to inject, 125, 125*f*, 126*f*
local anatomy for, 124
needle size/gauge for, 124
pitfalls/complications, 126
postinjection care, 126
Ultrasound with heat, 156

Vaccination, Hepatitis B, 3
Vasoconstrictor agents
CNS toxicity from, 11

Whiplash, 111
Wrist joint injection, 26, 29
CPT for, 26
examination findings prior to, 27
follow-up injections, 29
how and where to inject, 27, 28*f*
local anatomy, 27
medications to inject, 27
pitfalls/complications of, 27
postinjection care, 28

Xanthochromic fluid, 2*t*
X-rays
Acromioclavicular joint, 20
elbow, 26
glenohumeral joint, 18
wrist joint, 27

Yergason sign, 64

Z-joint injection, 193*f*, 194, 194*f*, 195*f*, 196*f*, 197*f*